CONQUERING
CHRONIC PAIN

CONQUERING
CHRONIC PAIN

SOLUTIONS AND STRATEGIES FOR PEOPLE WHO HAVE GIVEN UP HOPE

DR. WAYNE PHIMISTER

Conquering Chronic Pain: Solutions and Strategies for People Who Have Given Up Hope

Copyright © 2019 Wayne Phimister

BMD Publishing
All Rights Reserved

ISBN # 978-1722910662

BMD Publishing CEO: Seth Greene
Editorial Management: Bruce Corris
Cover Art & Layout: Kristin Watt

BMDPublishing@MarketDominationLLC.com
MarketDominationLLC.com

Printed in the United States of America

DEDICATION

To my wife Veronica, for all her unconditional love and support.

ACKNOWLEDGMENTS

First, I thank Seth Greene of Market Domination LLC, who inspired me to write my first book by interviewing leaders in the medical field, allied health care professionals and business people who have mastered pain. I thank his team for editing and organizing the interviews and transcripts for publishing, and for capturing my vision.

I give thanks to Britzie Suzie Solatorio, my virtual assistant in the Philippines who coordinates my activities online.

My deepest appreciation to the three most influential people in my life, my wife and parents. First my parents, William and Pat Phimister. For 18 years they raised me in a loving supportive family with my three sisters providing all the essential necessities to be successful in life. I thank you for your steadfast love from across the ocean in Scotland.

Finally, my dearest wife Veronica. Thank you for your endless love, support and commitment to follow my heart in the world of medicine, online business and writing this book. Through all lifes challenges, we have triumphed with 20 years of marriage and continue to move forward, stronger, wiser, and steadfastly in love. Thank you for always believing in my goodness, my heart, my purpose. We move on, with our four children, Orlagh, Celyne, Lachlan and Liam with love, compassion and gratitude leading the way.

INTRODUCTION

Every day, I hear heartbreaking stories of people suffering from chronic pain. Pain that keeps them from doing even the simplest things that so many people take for granted.

But I also hear stories of people getting their lives back from pain. Some of those people are my patients, who had given up hope before entering my office. There are millions more, around the world, who discovered that relief really can become reality.

Unfortunately, there are many, many more of the first group. As a doctor, I can only treat so many people. But as an educator, and an advocate, I can reach many more who still don't know about the effective pain management strategies that can help them make pain a thing of the past.

Which is why I chose to do this book. I too suffered from chronic pain. I too got my life back. Now I'm on a quest to help as many people around the world get the relief I know is possible, and which I provide to my patients.

These interviews will help do that. They're enlightening, even eye-opening. I'm grateful to those who so willingly shared their experience and expertise.

If you're suffering from chronic pain, or want to help those who are, get ready to learn about solutions and strategies.

More important, learn why pain doesn't have to be a life sentence.

Let's dive in, it's time to find pain solutions!

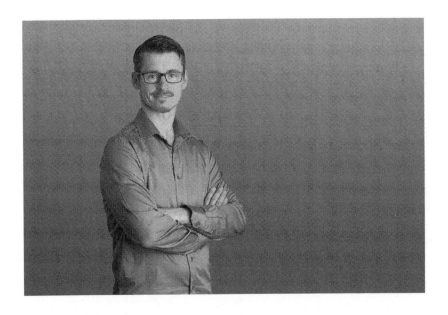

Dr. Wayne Phimister
May, 2019

TABLE OF CONTENTS

Chapter 1
WHO IS WAYNE PHIMISTER?

Pain. To me, it's a nasty four-letter word. And it's something that devastates people's lives. The people I interviewed for this book share that belief, and share my passion to help as many people as possible to reduce pain or live pain free, and live the type of life they deserve.

But before you hear from these amazing professionals, and get their insights on fighting and preventing pain, I'd like you to hear a little about me. Who is Dr. Wayne Phimister? How did I get here? Here meaning the Vancouver area in British Columbia, Canada, and also meaning this stage in my medical career, having this calling. In both cases, it's been quite a journey.

If you were hearing my voice, and my accent, you would know my journey started half a world away in Scotland. I grew up in a small town in the north of Scotland called Buckie. In high school I sparked an interest in sciences, and deep within me grew the desire to help people. This desire may come from my altruistic self or possibly from a near drowning accident when I was five years old, being rescued by a lifeguard. Whatever the reason, when I was a teenager I made the decision to turn those interests into a career in medicine. Then, when I was in medical school, I began planning a career in pediatrics. But in my final four weeks of medical school, my future became clear.

I was in a family doctor's office, and realized, "My goodness! This is where I need to be." It was like my heart was speaking to me. So off I went to be a family doctor.

But my life also had a few major changes coming. Years earlier, I had met a girl on vacation in Canada, and we became pen pals. In the passage of time, we became much more. We spent time together and realized we were meant for each other. She's been my wife ever since. She was from Vancouver, so we settled near her home in British Columbia. I put my Scottish medical degree to work, building a medical career in Canada.

My desires around family medicine led me into teaching, which was something I felt naturally inclined toward. I'm actually still teaching today. But my first desire was to help people. So I began practicing as a family doctor.

Then I had the realization that changed everything. It was about pain. I realized by focusing on that, I could help people who truly needed the help. People who were truly suffering. Most importantly, people who weren't being helped by "traditional" medicine.

So I began shifting towards a full time practice in pain management, and taking a more holistic approach. I trained in medical acupuncture and appreciated the role of balancing energy pathways in the body called meridians to achieve positive results in patients with chronic pain. In Vancouver, I trained with Dr. Chan Gunn and used his dry needling technique in daily family practice finding ways to release muscle tension and knots associated with pain. I then started doing trigger point injections, finding even better results treating painful muscles and painful areas of the body. And it built from there.

Which leads me to where I am today. I now work with teams of professionals in 3 clinics in the Vancouver area. We treat chronic pain from several different angles. My focus is trigger point injections, posture correction, cognitive approaches, and also the mind-body connection. That's where you realize the body is not just a mechanical entity but it's a physical form, with mental, emotional, and spiritual components. So I look at all these components as I try and help people with their daily struggles with chronic pain.

I like to say I specialize in giving people their lives back. It's heartwarming to me when I see them transforming, and having hope again. They're able to return to work, return to hobbies and activities they love. Many are able to get off the medications they've been taking for years. It's a real life-changing experience.

Let me tell you about one of those patients. A 65-year-old woman, I will call her Claire who was referred for chronic pain treatments as an amputee. She had lost a leg as a teenager and had suffered from chronic pain in her stump ever since. She had seen therapists, pain specialists, tried treatments and medications and nothing had worked. She was also slightly overweight and a type-one diabetic. I explained trigger point injections, and how they might help her, but I also focused on the mind-body approach. I advised her to read Dr. John Sarno's book, *Healing Back Pain,* which explains that we can direct our thoughts about pain to achieve a pain free live, and how we actually have more control over our pain than we think we do. It can be a very long journey towards healing our pain, or it can be very short for some people.

She took this message to heart, and within a handful of sessions she no longer had any pain in the stump. That was an amazing turnaround. Ten months later she's still pain free. She's a great advocate. She actually goes around the town in her wheelchair telling people about the mind body connection, and how pain is really embodied in our mind before it becomes embodied in our flesh. She's also lost over 40 pounds in weight with a plant-based diet and reversed the diabetic need for insulin all with the guidance of her own family physician. She's a great testimony to both the trigger point injections and the mind body connection. She is learning how to heal!

In many ways, she's both my ideal patient and my typical patient. Someone with chronic pain who's been through the system, has tried different types of doctors, different types of treatments, different types of medications, but still doesn't know why they're in pain and why they aren't getting better. They're fearful of the future. And they're open to the principles of how the mind and body work in unison.

Which is why a patient's first visit with me involves a full bio-psycho-social evaluation including a childhood history of trauma and abuse along with a physical examination. We then talk about treating pain in different ways with the body and mind, and explaining why the mind and the body are interconnected. So while I'm treating the pain in their body, we're working just as hard on their mind, reviewing where they're at and helping them move forward on their journey.

One of the reasons I'm so passionate about this, is because I also suffered from chronic pain. I also know what it's like to miss out on something that's important to you. When I was in my twenties, I suffered from chronic chest pain. It did not make sense, being a national level swimmer in my earlier days, I thought taking up running would be easy. I loved to do it. But the tightness across my chest was just too painful. I had to hang up my running shoes which crushed my spirit.

And no one knew why. I had medical test after test, and no one found the reason for my pain. But seven years later, I saw a Rolfing practitioner who did deep tissue massage, working her hands deep into my muscles and fascial tissue. And after 10 sessions, my pain was gone.

I was able to run again. Which gave me joy, and still does to this day. When I run, it makes my heart sing. I can get out there and detach from everything, and just be present with myself and my environment. It makes me feel whole.

Having this understanding of the muscle component of pain and the fascial component of pain led me to another major discovery, an "A-ha" moment if you will, a few years ago. I was treating patients with the dry needling technique using acupuncture needles into muscles that were tight and painful, something I had done for 12 years with great results. But I heard of other doctors using medical needles instead, so I tried that, and quickly discovered, "Wow, there's something else going on." I felt a resistance within the tissues. It was actually something I could hear and feel through the needle, and the patient could feel and hear it as well. It's actually a grinding noise. This grinding comes from blunting the needle as it penetrates the tissues. I soon learned, "Wow, this is fascia, this is a tight layer that is restricting tissues, restricting muscles, and is fundamental to the physical component of chronic pain conditions that people have."

From that moment on, I became even more passionate about finding pain solutions. If I could figure something out like that, and confirm it with my colleagues, there must be other novel ways of treating pain. That led me to an understanding about posture and the importance of posture alignment. Also, the mind-body connection, and through that, different cognitive behavioral techniques to optimize pain. So now I believe I'm on the path toward even more discoveries, and more solutions.

And I'm just thrilled to have a passion for reaching and teaching both patients and doctors about this simple trigger point injection technique that hardly anybody knows about. Unless you poke people with medical needles in this way, you're not going to understand this or know about it. So many family physicians and specialists are completely unaware of this.

Remember, for centuries, physicians have observed clinical findings from their patients and shared them with colleagues. Revolutionary medical breakthroughs have come by accident, such as, penicillin, which was discovered by the growth of mould on a petri dish inhibiting bacterial overgrowth. And look where we are today with treating infections. I believe my approach to trigger point injections is unique seeing the interconnected nature of the fascial tissue pivotal to unlocking the tightness in muscles and fascia throughout the body associated with chronic pain.

But the lack of knowledge about this is a huge frustration for me. I believe every family doctor who sees a patient in chronic pain could help at least half of them if they did trigger point injections understanding the role of tightened fascia and muscles.

There's so much that can be done very simply, if this was just common knowledge taught at medical school with its long lost physiological principle which describes nerves becoming super sensitized when they become traumatized. As doctors train and become specialized in one area or in general as family physicians the whole medical community would understand this very effective approach to treating pain.

Sadly, there's a divide between so-called traditional medicine and those who take a holistic approach. I myself say I have a holistic scientific practice, and there are those who would say that's an oxymoron.

I think the root of this is a 400 year old principle from René Descartes, the French philosopher who said we should study modern medicine through dualistic theory. That means you split the body into pieces, like the mind and the matter, or the mind and the body, or the body and all its different organs and systems. You split them up into different parts, and investigate them to find out what the problem is. We are still embodying this principle today.

The reality is we're not a human machine with parts. We are human beings with a body, mind, and spirit. Unless we start assessing patients as human beings and not human machines, this problem will not change. The question is whether we're willing to look at a person's body in its entirety with physical organs and tissues all interconnected with thoughts, emotions, beliefs, past and present experiences and environments. All these factors are influencing the current status of their health. The scientific research now backs this up.

Unfortunately, we still have a system where specialists are looking at one thing, whether it's the bones, the brain, the heart or any organ or part of the body, and not assessing how the mind effects it. Until we fully move to the theory of mind-body connection, we won't make real progress in treating chronic pain effectively.

My mission is to help 100 million people live pain free. Let me say that again. **Help 100 million people live pain free.** How can I possibly do that?

Certainly not by staying in my office poking people with trigger point injections. I need to share my voice, my story. I hope to teach around the world, and have access to Universities sharing my knowledge of why pain exists and how doctors can introduce my simple trigger point injection technique to their medical practice. When medicine encompasses the mind-body principle, integrating the advancements of neuroscience we shall see a shift in pain treatments.

I started teaching about 15 years ago, when I was working in New Zealand and had the opportunity to teach some medical students. I began with much anxiety and apprehension, but discovered I enjoyed it. When I first came to Canada, I was able to work with medical students and family medicine residents. Again, I enjoyed it. Then I taught behavioral medicine in the Department of Family Medicine at the University of British Columbia in Chilliwack. All of this broadened my insights on what is really needed to be a good teacher, which is to connect with your students, teach from first principles and relate to their journey of learning.

But you can only reach so many people in a classroom setting. Which is why I've moved to the online world. I've set up courses for trigger point injections and cognitive behavioral therapy that's very easily implemented by physicians who have an interest in this area. I'll be launching that soon.

Which leads me to this book. Why did I choose to do it, and why did I choose to talk to these people? When I realized there are treatment modalities out there that practitioners and physicians are using that actually work, I wanted to interview people who had come into this domain. None of us knows everything on how to treat chronic pain. There are many people out there who have successfully helped hundreds and thousands of patients. The book is my first round of interviews with people like physicians, pain doctors, therapists, psychiatrists and others who take a variety of different approaches.

I believe it will be a tremendous resource for patients with chronic pain, who have questions but aren't happy with the answers they've received, and aren't happy with their current treatments. If you're one of them, I think this will give you lots of different avenues to go down, and to learn so you become knowledgeable as well as successful in your approach to treating your pain condition.

My knowledge grew in leaps and bounds by doing these interviews. Some of them are also authors, and I'm reading their books. I'm also utilizing some of the techniques I've learned, and incorporating them into my practice. I just love learning, and I love having different ways of helping people.

Here's something important I've learned. Patients control their health. We, in the medical profession, must realize that physicians can help patients by dealing with their negative self-talk in their minds, and realize that healing is really an entity within us. If you break your arm, it heals. If you have a laceration on your skin, it heals. If you have a common cold, it heals. The same is true for many medical situations. And chronic pain is one of them.

When we can enter into a place of knowledge that the DNA in each of our 100 trillion cells are literally programmed to heal, and when we move into a mental space where we believe that and we can work on ourselves, with our therapists and our doctors together, supporting this principle, the power of the body is beyond what we really know and can imagine.

If we can just start the journey of believing that we can heal, then we will do amazing things in our journeys. As many of my patients have shown, it's really possible to heal from pain and the potential is there for other conditions too.

So let's start your journey now.

Chapter 2
TRIGGER POINT INJECTIONS

Trigger point injections (TPI) are an essential tool of the physician who successfully treats chronic pain. After 19 years of treating patients with acupuncture, then dry needling or intramuscular stimulation and now trigger point injections with lidocaine 1% solution, I have developed a winning formula to release pain and tightness in the body that accompanies chronic stress built up in the muscles, fascia and soft tissues.

The gold standard textbook for trigger point injections, *Myofascial Pain and Dysfunction: The Trigger Point Manual: Volume 1 and 2*, by Janet Travell and David Simons, highlights the standard trigger point injection release technique of myofascial knots that have characteristic referral patterns and jump responses when you inject these muscle knots. On page 18 of Volume 1, the authors allude to a more general muscle pain syndrome of any soft tissue that is associated with muscle tenderness. My experience has taught me that tightened fascia is the structure that holds physical pain within the soft tissues, such as muscles, tendons, ligaments, joint capsules and scars. Many people cannot find satisfactory results from physiotherapy, massage or chiropractic treatments but are effectively treated by inserting a medical hypodermic needle into the soft tissues by cutting small holes in the fascia, muscle and other tissues so releasing the tightness and freeing up movement and recovery for each part affected.

My practice has taught me that understanding the interconnected nature of fascia in the body that runs from head to toe around muscles, through muscles, connecting muscle to muscle, as well as around organs, and within tendons, ligaments and joint capsules is fundamental to optimally treating this tight layer. The peripheral nerves— which leave the spinal cord and travel to all areas of the body—get squished from this tightness leading to reduce blood flow of oxygen and nutrients which in turn cause hypersensitivity and pain.

An added complicated, often overlooked factor in the cause of chronic pain is the role of the autonomic nervous system (ANS) with psychological and emotional causes. The ANS has 2 parts—the sympathetic nervous system and parasympathetic nervous system. Both of these parts start in the limbic area of the brain and are distributed all around the body controlling cellular and tissue functioning. In chronic pain, the sympathetic nervous system is activated causing the commonly known flight-fight response or less commonly known stress response. This leads to muscle tension, tightness and reduced blood flow to the soft tissues affected.

Every day, with almost every patient I see, counting up to 150 per week have the same story of chronic pain, failed treatments, little understanding why chronic pain exists and a search for answers with successful treatments.

The understanding of peripheral nerve hypersensitivity and activation of the sympathetic nervous system is key to optimally treating chronic pain as shown by the co-authors in this book. Trigger point injections can kick start the healing response for a great number of people as shown by good—to—excellent response rate under my care when they complete 4-6 treatments.

In this book's second edition, I included this new chapter to share this essential knowledge for conquering chronic pain and offer new hope.

I interviewed three local colleagues in the Vancouver area. They have 26 years of experience, and have treated thousands of patients collectively with over 30,000 patients in their clinics with colleagues. They share the common results of transforming lives where people get their life back.

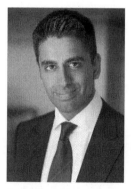

Dr. Ravi Dhanoa has been invited to speak on myofascial pain and trigger point injection therapy at many pain conferences at a regional and national level.

After opening a full service Family Practice on Vancouver Island, he trained in Trigger Point Injection therapy, developed his skills further through working as a pain clinic physician in Vancouver, and then opened The MuscleMD clinic in 2014.

Dr. Dhanoa is also Clinical Faculty at St Paul's Hospital, for the Family Medicine Residency Program at the University of British Columbia. He is involved in the training and assessment of

International Medical Graduates, Family Practice residents and medical students.

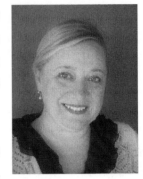

Dr. Inna Fadyeyeva provides Primary Dermatology services, and focuses on learning new ways of addressing skin issues with the use of newer technologies and natural remedies.

She received her medical degree from Kiev State Medical University, Ukraine, completed her Family Medicine Residency program at the University of British Columbia, and also completed the Cardiff Diploma Program in Practical Dermatology.

Dr. Fadyeyeva is a Clinical Instructor at the Department of Family Medicine UBC and enjoys teaching future generations of Family Physicians.

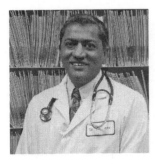

Dr. Minesh Naran believes he needs to inform and educate his patients first, and then guide them toward understanding and experiencing the benefits of exercise, nutrition and weight management in order to alleviate and manage pain.

Dr. Naran began his career practicing internal medicine at various hospitals in South Africa. He has had his own family practice in North Vancouver since 1993.

Dr. Naran obtained his Acupuncture qualification at the University of California, Los Angeles, and his certification in Trigger Point Therapy at George Washington University. He is affiliated with the College of Physicians and Surgeons in Canada, and a member of the Canadian Foundation of Acupuncture.

Trigger Point Injections: A Starting Point

Wayne: Ravi, you specialize in this specific form of pain treatment. What are trigger point injections?

Ravi: Essentially, it's a pretty well-established procedure, but it's not very well-known. It's been around since the 1960s, believe it or not. One of the first famous patients was JFK. It's been lost over the years, but more recently there's been a resurgence. It's a pretty simple procedure involving the injection of solution, which could be either a local anesthetic or saline or dextrose—which is sugar—or even Botox.

What you're doing is identifying areas of contracted muscle known as trigger points—which can cause characteristic pain patterns in the body or restriction in movement—and injecting a substance into the muscle, not always very deep. Hopefully, the action of the injection and the solution itself can help release the muscle from spasm and reduce the pain.

Wayne: Minesh, talk about how this technique works.

Minesh: This technique is mainly releasing the knots in the muscle. Most of the time—when it comes to pain—there are many diagnoses in western medicine. In this system, the theory is that most of pain in soft tissue origins is caused by muscles. If you can release or relax those muscles, you will decrease the pain and increase the movement.

Wayne: How common is it for people to have knots in their muscles?

Minesh: Very common. They're in almost every patient I see. It's just they're not diagnosed anymore by doctors, because they don't really know what it's all about. Nobody really looks for it; there's no imaging studies for trigger point therapy like MRI or X-Rays. Trigger points are found by manual therapy or by palpation.

Wayne: Inna, what type of conditions are you treating with trigger point injections?

Inna: I think it all started with tension headaches complaints from my patients, because it's such an overwhelming issue for a lot of people. I was quite frustrated, and that's where you, Wayne, came along. You basically said to me, "Well, there is a way to treat it without medication," which is quite effective. I tried it, it worked, and that was the beginning of really using the TPI. So, most of the patients I treat with trigger point injections have myofascial syndrome and are affected in different areas—mainly neck, upper back, lower back, and iliotibial band.

Finding Relief After Many Disappointments

Wayne: What treatments have these patients typically tried before?

Minesh: Oh, they've tried everything. They've tried medications, physiotherapy, massage therapy, chiropractic, acupuncture, exercise therapy, kinesiology... They've tried many, many things. Everybody's been around the block.

Wayne: Yes, and that's exactly what I find in my practice also. It's completely amazing. All of a sudden, when you insert the medical needle into those knots, you get a release. It's like a little bit of magic in the body.

Minesh: I've been called various names, and magician is definitely one of them.

Wayne: Inna, what other kinds of treatments have they tried?

Inna: Well, it really differs. Some people have been on different medications for many years. Others have tried acupuncture, physiotherapy, endless chiropractor visits, and massage therapy. For some people, it's sort of an acute phase, and they're quite desperate for pain medication. So, the first trial for them is typically to go on nonsteroidal anti-inflammatory medication. And some, unfortunately, go on opioids as well. Invariably, almost all of them are at the stage of desperation, because as we know, medications really don't help with this condition.

Wayne: What's your experience with these patients and what's actually going on in their bodies?

Inna: Again, the cases are quite different. Some have tension headaches and neck and upper back pain. For some people, it's way more complicated with fibromyalgia—non-diagnosed or diagnosed—where the body aches are overwhelmingly everywhere in different places at different times. These people have real issues pinpointing where their main area of concern is. You start focusing on what's the most troubling or most difficult for them at the time, and then you move from one area to the other.

Wayne: Could you describe a scenario for me? Say a patient has low back pain with referral pain down their leg to the ankle. It's not a slipped disc compressing the sacral nerve—which we can sometimes diagnose on examination and then confirm on CAT scan or MRI scan—but actually it's the tightened fascia compressing the peripheral nerves. I'm sure some readers have experienced low back pain going down their leg, and they're convinced they have sciatic nerve compression in their lower back. However, their scans are normal and are left with the question, "Well, what's going on?"

Ravi: Absolutely. This is something we see at my clinic on a daily basis. Pain down the leg doesn't necessarily mean—as you said—sciatic nerve compression.

Now, by the time patients come into our clinic, we usually have the benefit of imaging—meaning the patient either had a CAT scan or an MRI scan— because their physician sees them and says, "Well, look. This sounds like sciatica. Go and get physio, etc." Things don't get better, even though they've been doing everything they're meant to do to treat the sciatic nerve. Then they get a CAT scan or an MRI, and it comes back and everything is absolutely fine.

In these instances, they're can be a number of things causing lower back pain. A lot of the times it comes down to the fascia, usually in the lumbosacral region—meaning just above the buttock area of the lower back. Very superficially treating that area can resolve a lot of this pain. Also, when the gluteal muscles are tight, they cause pain that travels down the leg. Patients may not necessarily notice that they have tight muscles in their buttock area. However, once the area's treated, they often find that things resolve. When we apply pressure to these areas, over the muscle and the fascia only, patients will feel that characteristic radiation of pain that does shoot down the leg.

So often we do see this being the case, and patients respond very well. However, the caveat is: many people can have pathology in their backs. They can have a slipped disc, or they can have tight muscles and have fascial injury. You can go for surgery; you can have a neurosurgeon fix the back and do a perfect job, and the patient will come out and still have the pain, which—according to the surgeon—will make no sense, because they'll have had imaging after the procedure and the surgeon will say, "Well, look. Everything looks great. The nerves aren't being pinched anymore. So, I'm not quite sure why you have pain. Maybe you should go and get some physiotherapy and that'll do the trick." However, quite often it's the fascia that's injured.

Success Stories

Wayne: There are many people who live with chronic pain who think, "I'm in pain, and I've tried lots of things. I've been to the physiotherapist, the chiropractor, the massage therapist and acupuncturist and it's just not working." Please share a story where you helped a patient with trigger point injections.

Ravi: I've been treating a woman in her 40s who's been suffering with migraine headaches for the longest time. The headache starts at the back of the head. She feels tightness in the neck, and the pain shoots forward. In describing the pain behind her eyes, she feels like there's a pressure sort of pushing her eyes outwards when she has these headache episodes.

She'd been to her family doctor. She had a scan of her head to make sure there's no space-occupying lesion—meaning there's something in there that shouldn't be that's causing an increase of pressure inside the cranium. Of course, everything was clear. She's been trialed on multiple medications.

At first, it didn't make any sense to her, but I started examining her neck and her shoulder muscles. She said, "Well, I don't have any pain in my shoulders." Then, you sort of press on the muscles around the trapezius—which is the broad muscle that goes across the upper back—and naturally, she has tight areas there. We refer to those as trigger points. When I was pressing on certain areas in the trapezius muscle and then to the muscle known as the splenius capitus, I was able to recreate that exact headache pain that she experiences.

So just by physically pushing with my fingers in certain areas, I gave her the headache that she usually experiences momentarily. Since I could identify those as being the causes for her headache, over the last few treatments we've had great success in reducing the frequency.

Wayne: Minesh, what are your results with these treatments?

Minesh: 70% to 80% of the patients I treat will find some form of relief with this therapy. I tell patients to try at least four treatments and see how they do. I tell them, "If this treatment is good for you, within four treatments you should be at least 40% better." Not everyone reaches that threshold, but at least 70% to 80% of patients feel somewhat better.

Wayne: Inna, can you share a specific case story that would inspire people to try trigger point injections?

Inna: A 77-year-old woman was referred to me by another physician. She presented with restless leg syndrome, and a five-year history of not sleeping at night because of the restlessness she felt in her left leg. She had seen at least three different neurologists. She did EMG studies. She had seen a physiatrist, a rheumatologist, and internal medicine professionals. She was at the end of her rope. She said, "I don't care what you do. If you can do even a little bit for me, I would be grateful."

In these situations, you can't really over promise anything, because you don't know how they're going to react. So I basically suggested to try it without any promise at all. She did have a sensitive left iliotibial band on exam all the way down to her ankle. We started doing weekly sessions, using a 50/50 mixture of normal saline and lidocaine. Within three weeks, she started sleeping at night. That was a really dramatic case for me, because I didn't expect her to improve so quickly.

We've now been doing weekly trigger point injections for six months. She's sleeping at night. Her upper leg has no symptoms at all. She has a bit of discomfort in her lower leg and more discomfort in her foot, but overall, she rates her improvement as 65-70%.

Is she very happy? Absolutely. Would she be happier if she had zero symptoms? Absolutely. However, I think realistically somebody who is 77 will not be able to have their symptoms 100% removed. There is arthritis present, and her general muscular condition is not the best.

Still, that case was incredible for me, because I just could not believe that the effect of the very simple procedure could have such a profound effect on her function and life. As you can imagine, she was completely exhausted mentally, emotionally, and physically from not sleeping at night for five years. Now, she's coming back to life, and she's doing activities she has not done for years.

Moving Forward

Wayne: What's your hope for the future of this type of treatment?

Inna: I hope more family physicians would incorporate their approach to musculoskeletal issues with trigger points, and not be afraid to actually start using this technique. I think it's doable. Everyone who has come through our clinic is already aware, and I think there are more people out there who are aware. I hope patients will ask their doctors, "Could I have that at your place as well?"

I think it's doable, and I'm really encouraged by you, Wayne. You've been a promoter of this technique, and it definitely changed my practice. It changed my life as a patient, and I hope it happens for many other people.

Wayne: What's the biggest challenge you are faced with now?

Minesh: I think the main challenge is to let all other practitioners know that these modalities exist. As more practitioners become aware, they can start practicing it in their own practice, because most of them have lidocaine available to them quite easily in their offices. Once this technique is learned, they can start relieving their patients' pain much faster.

Wayne: As you move forward treating people with trigger point injections, what advice would you have for your patients, and other people out there who are in pain?

Ravi: I think the most important thing for patients to do is to become aware of their body. Become aware of what their symptoms are, and what causes symptoms. When you know the cause, that's the way you can resolve pain. It's not always a simple medical solution. We always look for a quick fix. My advice to all patients—and this is after being a physician for quite a while—is, "let's try and avoid the medication approach if we can, because that's a slippery slope in many cases."

When you have chronic pain, it's very easy to fall into dependency on medications. These days, more and more people are stepping away from the narcotic medications and muscle relaxants. Sometimes, those medications are great in a pinch or emergency, but all too often we become reliant on them and think we can't manage without them. The more pain killers we use the more we need them. That's the danger.

I always say to patients, "if there's one less person out there that is taking medications as a result of treatment, I feel like I've done a good job as a physician." That's my big take home message.

This chapter contains just a portion of the interviews I did with these three doctors. You can hear the entire interviews on my podcast. There's a link to that on my website: https://waynephimister.com/podcast/

They shared a lot of new information about this growing pain-relief treatment. I hope you are inspired to seek out a physician in your area who does this technique.

Chapter 3
KELSEY BAAS

Dr. Kelsey Baas holds a Doctorate in Physical Therapy. She is the owner and physical therapist at *Compleo Physical Therapy & Wellness* in Woodland, Texas, where they utilize a multi-disciplinary approach to pain. In 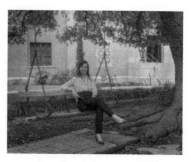 addition to physical therapy, Compleo also offers a licensed professional counselor and a registered dietitian.

Dr. Bass previously served as a clinical specialist and the Chronic Pain Clinic physical therapist at Texas Children's Hospital.

She is also BSPSTS Certified, a Schroth-based treatment method for scoliosis.

Wayne: Dr. Kelsey Baas is a doctor of physical therapy. After working at a pediatric chronic pain clinic, she has her own clinic in Texas, where she helps both children and adults with pain management strategies. Kelsey, thank you for being here. Let's go back in time. Where did you grow up and what was your childhood like?

Kelsey: I grew up in Dallas, Texas. The Lone Star State. It's a great place. I had a great childhood, a typical childhood. I loved my family, and grew up with both my parents and my sister. I was very involved in ballet all the way through my childhood. And that's really what got me my passion for movement and led me to the physical therapy. I love to move and help other people move, and if you're hurting a lot you're not able to do that. So from a young age I started to appreciate the importance of movement.

Wayne: Yes, I can relate to that. As a family physician who focuses his practice on helping patients find solutions for chronic pain, I realize the role of movement is absolutely essential. However, when patients are in pain, their bodies often tighten up, so we have to overcome that as well as treat the pain.

It's great you chose a training path involving pediatrics, a very unique area in the pain world. Please tell us how you came to train in traditional physical therapy, and where you are right now?

Kelsey: As you said, I started in traditional physical therapy school. I got my undergraduate with the basic science anatomy prerequisites, and went on to get my doctorate of physical therapy at UT Southwestern, which was a fantastic education. I really feel the most important thing about my graduate program is they taught me how to think critically, and they gave me the pure basis of movement. I learned it's up to us to continue to apply that critical thinking as your career progresses, as new evidence comes out.

I do a lot of things the same way I was taught in school, but there are a lot of things I do differently based on new articles and new things I've learned. That was a more traditional physical therapy model. Then, during my time at Texas Children's Hospital, I had the honor of serving on quite a few multi-disciplinary teams from lung transplant to chronic pain, and really saw the value of multiple disciplines coming together. From physicians to psychologists, we all bring something unique to the table, and I think we're best as a team.

That's where I started to really appreciate the multi-disciplinary model. I also went to a pain neuroscience education course with Dr. Adrian Lowe, who really got me thinking about the mind-body connection a little more, a little past just the musculoskeletal system. I started to really see the value in the combination of psychology and physical therapy, especially with pain. That's what led my interest to participation in our chronic pain clinic at Texas Children's, and now here in Waco involving psychology in my physical therapy practice.

Wayne: Wonderful story. Now you have your own clinic, and have other therapists with their particular focus of practice. You mentioned a psychologist and I know you have a dietician also. Tell us how that actually works. When you assess a new patient, do all three disciplines work closely together?

Kelsey: It's really patient specific. Some patients need all three disciplines, some just need one. The most common combination is physical therapy and psychology. But there is so much floating around on doctor Google about anti-inflammatory diets, or the Keto diet, so the dietitian is there to answer those questions. I think from the dietitian's standpoint, patients come in wanting to try all these extreme things, so it's actually made their life more stressful. She can calm them down and say, "Okay, maybe let's talk about decreasing sugar. That can affect our body and how we feel. But we don't need to cut out everything we love."

When I evaluate a patient, or do what's called a discovery visit where they come to see the clinic, I look at how they're moving. We talk about their history, how long they've been in pain, and we go into psychosocial stressors like anxiety and life at home. I can pretty quickly get a feel for what is contributing to their pain and their stress. Unfortunately, a lot of them have been through past traumas that they've never really managed or dealt with. It's so sad that we weren't able to give them the tools earlier. It's like their body can only take holding that in for so long.

We recommend that all of our chronic pain patients get at least an evaluation with counseling and physical therapy. Then as a team we decide how much of each that patient really needs. It's nice to work together and be in the same building. Say the counselor is working with pain coping strategies. When they come to physical therapy, if we're trying movement they haven't tried in a while, we have the option to bring the counselor in and walk them through those pain coping strategies while we're getting them up and walking again, which is really neat.

Wayne: Excellent. What would be your ideal type of client?

Kelsey: Like I said, I was at Texas Children's Hospital before, so I love working with adolescents and children. I love to have a variety. I don't get bored if I have several of one age, but I like the variety of ages. However, for an ideal client, I'd say teenagers and young adults. They just provide a different challenge. Especially the teenagers, where you get to work with the whole family and not just the patient. I love solving puzzles that haven't been solved yet. Unfortunately I get to do that because many of my patients have already been to many providers and haven't gotten any answers. But I love to get that challenge, and get to dig a little deeper, and hopefully be the one who is able to get them back to function.

Sometimes I hesitate to say pain free in my chronic pain world. We really focus on function and try not to ask what their pain level is. That's why I say I like to be the one to get them back to function. But I really like the complicated cases. The ones that are a puzzle, I love that.

Wayne: I completely relate to that. Let's consider a patient you recently treated. Obviously we won't mention any names, but share how you were able to help them and really make a big difference.

Kelsey: I've had a young pediatric client. Younger than a teenager. The family came in really discouraged. Out of nowhere, he started having this pain that completely took him out of sports. He's a really active, amazing kid, and it's so hard to have to watch one like that just sit on the sidelines. He went to a couple other therapists where he failed treatment, and actually got a little bit worse. But after coming through the clinic and using some of the graded motor imagery techniques, working laterality, things like that, we've made progress.

This week we have him walking with a shoe on again. We all take that for granted, but for him that was a huge accomplishment. The first couple visits he had to be carried in, or crutch in. To see him walking in with his shoes on, and getting closer to being back on the soccer field, has been really rewarding this month.

Wayne: Wow, that's wonderful. When you're treating clients, what are the specific treatment modalities you use to help them move forward?

Kelsey: A lot of things. Again, it's very patient dependent. There's no kind of "one prescription fits all," but definitely a lot of manual myofascial work. Really working with the fascia system, which is in between the skin and the muscles. That takes a lighter touch than the deep tissue trigger point release. We do go into the more muscular releases, but a lot of patients can't tolerate that type of touch.

I had one patient come to me whose therapist had been dry needling, and it was sending her autonomic nervous system into almost even more panic, and she was having crazy reactions. We start with the fascial system, and a much lighter touch than what you would think of for a myofascial release. So many therapists now are doing the dry needling, which for a non-chronic pain population is fantastic, or for a patient who can tolerate that type of pressure can be great.

We do a lot of education. We spend lots of time educating on central sensitization. I have to credit Dr. Adrian Lowe for this analogy, but really talking about your nervous system as an alarm system, and how the sensitivity is turned up. It's like if a leaf would blow by our house alarm and set the alarm off, instead of the alarm only going off when someone breaks in. We do a lot of desensitization work, exposing patients to different temperatures, pressures and textures, so they can get used to typical sensations again. Putting tags in their clothes, those types of things.

Of course, I'm a physical therapist, so movement is a big part. We assess posture. We assess their quality of movement. I try hard to focus on functional movements and how they're performing those. It's great if you can sit on a table and turn on the muscle, but if that doesn't carry over to squatting to pick up your child, or your toys at home, that doesn't really do that much. We really work on how they are performing functional movements, and what asymmetries we see in that, and how can we fix that so those movements are a little bit less painful.

Those are some of the things we start with, and then we do some motor imagery, progressive relaxation techniques in the chronic pain population. Then, from there, it just really depends on the patient. Sometimes we'll put a TENS on but not that often.

Wayne: You're very aware of how the body essentially gets stuck in one position, or one area, and whether it be the posture or their muscles, or around the muscles in the fascial layer, which is connecting all of the body together from top-to-toe. I find exactly the same thing.

I can relate to what you're saying, and I've also learned a few things. Thank you for that.

On a different note, what's the best advice you've ever received?

Kelsey: I have received a lot of good advice. I actually think the best advice I ever received was from my pediatrician when I was in high school, and I was thinking about going to physical therapy school. When I was talking about what my undergraduate degree might be in, she said, "To be a good healthcare practitioner, you have to be a really well rounded person. And you're going to be learning the rest of your life. If you're not learning the rest of your life, you're a bad practitioner." She told me I shouldn't major in a healthcare-related field, I should major in something that was going to make me well rounded. Then she said, "It's just great to study for the sake of studying."

I majored in Spanish, which has actually been a great skill I've gotten to use in the healthcare field, especially in Texas. When I was in a hospital system, we had a lot of Spanish speaking patients. Communicating with the patient is the most important thing. If I hadn't gotten that advice, I don't think I ever would have chosen to major in Spanish. I would have chosen something like biology or PT. That definitely has contributed to me being a more well-rounded person and set me up for the expectation to be a good practitioner. Not only do I need to learn my whole life but look outside of our traditional medical model. To approach the whole person.

Wayne: That's beautiful. Now that you have your own clinic, what's the biggest challenge you're facing?

Kelsey: Our clinic has only been open a couple months, so there are a couple challenges. One, we are not your traditional clinic setup, and I think especially for the city we're in, everything we're doing is very new. The PT counseling combination is very new. A lot of physicians still want to just go straight to medicines or injections. I can think of one patient in particular who's been struggling with back pain for a while. His doctor told his mother to just try heat and Tylenol a little longer.

We're talking about an epidemic of opioids in our country. And from a young age, if we're teaching children just to pop pills for their pain, even if it is just starting as a Tylenol, what could that be in 20 years if we're not teaching them how to manage that? I'd like to see other healthcare providers see this as a first line, instead of patients having to find us. Just about all my patients have found me, which is great that they've been able to do the research, but how many more patients could we be touching if as a community we had physicians buying into referring to this model of care? That has definitely been a challenge.

The other big challenge is, I have a huge heart and I really want to help all these adults and kids. But it's expensive if you're not under the umbrella of a big system. We need to be able to keep our doors open and provide the resources our patients need, and that we feel are best for the patient, but we have to match that with a price point that is affordable for the patient. Because, if you think about someone in pain, they have been to so many doctors. If it's an adult, many have had to miss work. So saying, " I think this is going to help, but you have to pay out of pocket for this PT and counseling," is a huge barrier for a lot of patients.

So as we are getting our feet wet as a new clinic, and facing challenges, that has also been a challenge for our clients.

Wayne: Thank you for that. Let's change the direction a little bit. You mentioned how counseling can help your pediatric and adult population. How does that work in reality?

Kelsey: There are a couple different avenues our counselor works in. One, which you mentioned you do as well, is cognitive behavioral therapy, CBT. The program our counselor went through does a lot of that, so she's able to work with that and the clients. I mentioned a lot of patients have undergone past traumas, so it's important to help them deal with and cope with whatever traumas or psychosocial stressors are going on in their lives. Pain can come with depression. If you're having to sit out of activity every day, imagine how you would feel. None of us feel good when we are sick and spend a day on a couch, so imagine having spent a year sitting on the sidelines, or PE, or having to leave school early all the time, or work early.

I have found there is definitely a connection between mood and how they perform in physical therapy. So we work to bring their anxiety down. They haven't moved in so long, some are really scared to move. We give them coping strategies they can work with for the anxiety. It can range from what you think of as typical counseling, depression, anxiety, to CBT and graded motor imagery, those types of pain coping techniques.

Wayne: Thank you for that. One final question, where can people find out more about your clinic and about what you do?

Kelsey: They can look us up online, compleowaco.com, or they can call us at 254-892-4957.

Wayne: Thank you Dr. Kelsey Baas for this interview. It's been fascinating.

Chapter 4
PETER BRESLIN

Peter Breslin, MD, is a psychiatrist
with a private practice in Richmond,
Virginia, which utilizes an eclectic and
teamwork-driven approach to
optimize their patients' well-being.

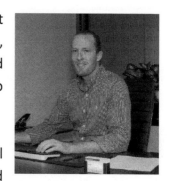

Dr. Breslin offers services in general
psychiatry, addiction psychiatry, and
forensic psychiatry.

He was chosen by his colleagues and peers as a *Richmond
Magazine Top Doc* in both Addiction Medicine and Adult
Psychiatry.

Wayne: Dr. Peter Breslin is a psychiatrist who specializes in
           addiction and psychiatry. Dr. Breslin, thank you for
           joining me. Let's start by going back to your
           childhood. Where did you grow up?

Peter: I grew up in northern Virginia. I lived there until I was
           just out of college. After that I went to medical
           school in the Caribbean, and then I did my residency
           in psychiatry at Virginia Commonwealth University,
           here in Richmond. I got to really enjoy Richmond.
           I've noticed as other colleagues move back to their

hometowns they find it difficult to start practices, and network. One of the advantages I had coming here for a residency was knowing the territory and a lot of the resources, which was really helpful for me.

Wayne: What made you specialize in addictions and psychiatry?

Peter: There's a long-winded answer to that, but the shortened version would be just the reciprocity of being able to help people. In a lot of psychiatry, you kind of beat yourself up a lot of times, because it's really difficult to help some people at times. In the field of addiction, when somebody comes in saying that they have a problem, It's nice to be able to grab it, work with it, and be able to turn it around and say, "Okay, if you're coming in with a history of opioid dependence but you have this chronic pain, we need to tease these things apart, and we need to find ways to manage a lot of these things with as little opioid as possible." Then I can easily work with that, and patients are usually highly motivated. So let's say there's also a good motivation factor when you're working in this field.

Wayne: So what is one of the best things about being in this field for you?

Peter: It never ceases to amaze me how people get better, get their lives back, and get into a better place.

Especially in addiction, because people are often at their last resort, and at the bottom of where they ever could imagine where they would be. I get to take that and get them back to where they were. It's one of the most amazing feelings I've had in this whole field. It's interesting, males and females have different kind of things. For example, a man will have sold his car, sold everything he has. And one of the biggest factors at first is when he can say, "Man I've got a car again, finally." It's almost like one of those rites of passages coming back, as they get back into a more functional world. It's very rewarding to a large degree.

Wayne: Wonderful. I can relate to helping patients turn their life around and really progressing towards a new life. It's just fantastic. What are the common questions people ask you when they see you?

Peter: Generally people want to know background. They want to know if I personally have a history of addiction. I think it's one of those sizing-up things, but also more importantly, I think it's an empathy thing. A lot of times people do addiction work without much understanding of what that person struggles with or is going through. I think what patients are looking for is someone able to understand and empathize, and not just judge them. I think that's one of the problems with addiction, there's too much judgment. I don't think it's addictionologists that are judging, I think it's a lot of the other fields. But I can't be too negative about it, because that ER doctor that continually sees a person coming in for this pain, and is having to treat them, may not feel they're doing right by the patient by giving them opiates, but that's the only thing that will help them in the moment. To me, the biggest thing is being able to sit down and work with these people so they feel that they're being heard and understood.

Wayne: I can see that. What specific techniques do you use to help patients with stress or to induce relaxation? Is that a part of your practice?

Peter: Yes, actually that's one of the more interesting things, as people get out of that first stage of withdrawals, is trying to deal and cope with stress and life. I hate to be pessimistic, but my view of American life is that it's just overwhelming. It's so much for a human to navigate and deal with. So I have a good number of nurse practitioners who have this as their main focus. How do we help these people? Whether it's somebody getting back into the gym and getting things kick started, because I feel exercise is a big part of stress management. Whether it's something like CBT and dealing with anxiety, because a lot of people get addicted due to either anxiety or depression. Therapy absolutely has to be a huge component of getting better.

And then you have some more simple things, like recovery groups and AA. Those are good, but it can be hit or miss for a lot of people, when it comes to those meetings. I prefer something that's a little bit more tailored to the person. So we continually work on resources for people so they have the highest chance of doing well.

Wayne: I love your approach to stress management, it's great. Thanks for sharing.

Can you tell us about a recent patient you treated, keeping it confidential? What was the situation, and how did they come through that experience?

Peter: I work largely with a recovery group called the McShin Foundation in Richmond, which has helped countless people and their families. McShin is a large organization. It's incredibly intimidating. People have to interact with people in large groups, and they have to do readings and stuff like that. It's really, really stressful for a lot of people who have a baseline level of anxiety. So just being able to work with them, even if it means having to go to a meeting or something like that, to help people feel more comfortable, or helping them get to know the other staff. Because once people realize that not everybody is against them, and they're actually trying to help them, it's a completely different kind of catalyst that happens. So just making people feel welcome, honestly.

Wayne: Who would be an ideal patient for you?

Peter: I really don't think there is such a thing as an ideal patient. Everybody comes from a different turmoil of life. Sometimes I have a little bit stronger of an empathy with certain struggles they've gone through. But it really doesn't change any part of my treatment plan, because there honestly is no typical patient. A lot of people have had a similar history, but everybody is so completely unique.

Wayne: I agree. So what's the biggest challenge you're facing right now in your career?

Peter: What I'd eventually like to do is go from a small office with therapists and providers, to something that's more encompassing. Maybe even like a rehab one day. It would take an incredible amount of work, because now you're dealing with different types of insurances and it becomes a logistical nightmare. I think this is one of the hard parts that not many people realize, the back-end work involved in trying to get people help. It isn't as much medicine as it is almost a business.

And it's sad, because you have to navigate these insurance companies and make sure that things get paid for. Career-wise, that's probably my biggest challenge. Being able to navigate the healthcare system. I get why patients are so frustrated with the healthcare system, because it's so incredibly confusing, and I don't feel it's 100% there to really help people all the time. Yes, ERs are wonderful and stuff like that, but once you get into a health insurance company putting up prior authorizations and blocking care, and things like that, you need a whole team of people to navigate something like that.

Wayne: Is there something you'd like to share that I haven't already asked you?

Peter: I have a really strong opinion of addiction. The thing I would hope you could pass along is trying to have family members really understand their kids, their loved ones, and not just have such a negative opinion. Because these negative opinions about addictions just make things worse. It doesn't help people. Loved ones need support, not judgment. Because recovery won't get off the ground unless that person has support and love in their life. There are cases where people do get better, but it's far and few between without loved ones.

Wayne: It's true. It takes a community to raise an individual. And it takes a community to help an individual move forward with their struggles, their addictions and their problems.

Where could people go to learn more about you or your services?

Peter: As you know, my practice is in Richmond, Virginia. My website is peterbreslinmd.com. I'm also trying to start a rebrand. I want to start a practice called Verity Addiction, and grow from there, and try to help as many people as possible.

Wayne: Thank you for sharing this information. I wish you the very best in this endeavor, and to your new vision of helping more and more people.

Chapter 5

DAVID CLARKE

David D. Clarke, MD is President of the *Psychophysiologic Disorders Association*, which works to advance the diagnosis and treatment of stress-induced medical conditions. He is also Assistant Director at the Center for Ethics and Clinical Assistant 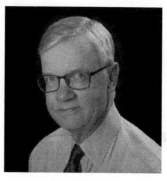 Professor of Gastroenterology Emeritus at Oregon Health & Science University in Portland, Oregon.

Dr. Clarke has conducted detailed interviews with over 7,000 patients whose pain or other symptoms were not explained by diagnostic tests. He summarized his findings in his book, *They Can't Find Anything Wrong!*

Dr. Clarke has been a Visiting Professor at Oxford University in England and the Royal Children's Hospital in Brisbane, Australia. He lectures about psychophysiologic disorders to health care professionals and the public across North America and in Europe.

Wayne: Dr. David Clarke is a gastroenterologist specializing in the diagnosis and treatment of illness linked to various forms of stress. He's very well known in the field of psychophysiologic disorders. Dr. Clarke, thank you for being interviewed. Let's start with your medical education.

David: I went to the University of Connecticut, School of Medicine, and followed that up with Harbor UCLA Medical Center for my residency and fellowship.

Wayne: Did you go directly into gastroenterology?

David: Yes, I'm very traditionally trained. I really had no idea back then that I was going to become so involved with psychophysiologic disorders. In fact, two thirds of my practice was very normal gastrointestinal work, putting endoscopes inside people, stopping hemorrhaging, removing gallstones, biopysing tumors, that sort of thing. But the other third of my practice, which has totaled over 7,000 patients, were people whose symptoms were not explained by diagnostic tests.

Wayne: How did you find yourself taking an interest in the mind component of illness?

David: It really started with one patient who had been severely ill for a couple years. She was a woman in her mid-30s who came to us at UCLA where I was in training. We had some very specialized testing which turned out to be normal, just like all her other tests. I accidentally uncovered the fact that she had been under a severe amount of stress. I didn't know what to do with that information at the time, but there was a psychiatrist there at UCLA, Harriet Kaplan, who became something of a mentor for me.

She was able to cure that patient with counseling alone in less than three months, which was remarkable to me. Nothing in my training up to that point even indicated such a thing was possible. So I decided, "You know, I should learn something about this, since it will likely come up, perhaps a few times a year." Then, when I got into practice, I found out it was a few times a week, then it was five or six times a week, and then I was doing 90% of the second opinions for my department of 12 other gastrointestinal physicians. It just kind of exploded from there.

Wayne: What would you say your biggest challenge is in this field?

David: There are a lot of challenges. The clinical challenge is to uncover the psychosocial stress a particular patient is struggling with. The reason this has been so much of a blind spot in the healthcare system, falling in between the expertise of both medical and mental health professionals, is that many patients can't articulate the real stress they're struggling with. So that's the clinical challenge.

The system challenge is to try to get the healthcare system to recognize that this condition exists, that psychosocial stresses of various kinds are fully capable of causing real symptoms that can be every bit as severe as those caused by organ diseases or structural abnormalities. And then to change the system so it involves medical and mental health professionals in an integrated way in the delivery of care.

That's what I've spent most of the last 10 years trying to do. Educate healthcare professionals on both sides of the mind/body divide to try to work together to produce better outcomes for these patients, which is eminently possible. The difficult clinical situations these patients present can be diagnosed and treated every bit as successfully as organ diseases and structural abnormalities.

Wayne: That's certainly something I've come to realize in my practice also. The more we dive into this world of mind-body connection, the more you realize solutions exist. There are options and treatments that can really benefit patients.

Say a patient with chronic abdominal pain comes in to see you. What are you looking for in this patient? What kind of questions are you asking them?

David: I do what I call a Stress Evaluation. That has six parts to it. It starts with an evaluation of the patient's chronology of their symptoms, when and where they started, and what their progress has been over time. Then I look to see, is the person under stress at the moment? Is there something going on in their life right now that's a challenge for them?

A subset of that is, are they the kind of person that takes care of everybody else in their world but has difficulty putting themselves on the list of people they take care of? These are folks that, if they get five or 10 minutes of free time, they start looking around for something useful and constructive they can do rather than something enjoyable for themselves. After a while, that lifestyle can catch up with you and the body starts to protest.

But probably the single biggest area I look into is whether the individual experienced stress as a child. Probably the most straightforward summarizing question there is whether the individual went through experiences growing up that they wouldn't want their own children to go through. This can be out and out abuse, it can be lack of support, it can be neglect, it can be never feeling like anything you did was good enough for your parents, it can be bullying at school, violent neighborhoods, substance abuse by the parents, a death or imprisonment or divorce, or any other form of loss of a parent. Any of a variety of negative experiences people can have growing up can have a long-term impact that can last decades into adulthood. There are all kinds of personality characteristics from people who emerged from those environments and physical symptoms as well.

Then, the final three areas I look into are garden variety mental health conditions that can be missed by the healthcare system because they present themselves to the system, not as a mental health issue, but as a physical symptom. Depression does this commonly, post-traumatic stress does this commonly, and the anxiety disorders do this commonly. A person goes to the doctor, tests are done, and nothing shows up. But the individual doesn't feel that depressed. They don't necessarily feel that anxious, and they may not connect their symptoms with the trauma they went through when they have PTSD. So it's very easy for a physician who's not clued into this to miss it completely.

Wayne: That's right. So you've done your stress evaluation questionnaire, and you dive in with more questions. You're getting to know your patient, you're connecting with them, and building rapport. Then, you perform a clinical exam. How valuable is that exam?

David: You always want to do the diagnostic tests and the physical exam that are necessary to be sure there's no organ disease nor structural abnormality. The stress factor certainly doesn't rule out an ulcer or a gallstone or a tumor, so we need to make sure those things are not present.

Some of the clues I get from the physical exam that it's stress related are when the symptom is located in a very small area. Most abdominal pain that's coming from something inside the abdomen tends to be smeared out over a fairly broad area because, as you know, the number of neurons inside the abdomen are relatively sparse and you can't get a precise signal about where the pain is coming from. So when a patient tells me their pain is coming from an area that's the size of a silver dollar for example, which I see fairly commonly, that's not likely to be coming from something inside the abdomen. So that's a clue.

Another clue the physical exam can give you is when the patient is telling you the symptom is very severe. They're desperate, they can't take the pain anymore, they're begging you to do something for them. But on the physical exam I'm not finding very much in terms of severity. Particularly if I examine that area and then other areas, and then come back to the painful area and I find it's just not that severely tender. That's a clue that this is probably stress related.

Wayne: So you've taken a comprehensive history, you've examined the patient, and you've done your tests, which come back negative. You haven't identified anything organic or physical. Then you move on to treatment. What options are you providing your patients?

David: We want to tailor the treatment to the specific stress or stresses the individual is suffering from. Here's a simple example. If they're in a domestic violence situation and it has been going on for a period of time corresponding to the length of time of the symptoms, then it's pretty clear that we need to do something about that relationship, or the symptoms are going to continue.

A more complex situation is the individual who is experiencing the long-term impact of stress from when they were children. There are a number of interventions we want to do there, starting with helping people recognize they've truly done a heroic thing by having survived that early adversity. One of the long-term impacts of what we call ACEs, or adverse childhood experiences, is impact on your self-esteem, making you feel like you're a second-rate human being.

I want people to realize that actually, the opposite is the case. To me, somebody who's been through that kind of experience and who's survived it and made a life for themselves, fits the definition of a hero. A hero is somebody who's overcome a difficult physical or mental challenge for a good cause. I don't want people to think of themselves as second-rate or somehow less worthy than other people. I want them to see they've really done something truly remarkable. They didn't wind up in that childhood adversity through any fault of their own, but they deserve a lot of credit for having come through that and survived it and made something of themselves in spite of it. So, helping change that self-image is a key foundation.

If they are having difficulty with their self-care skills, if they're not somebody that knows how to take a break or do something enjoyable on a regular basis, I want them to learn that skill. That turns out to be something essential for human beings to know, to set aside the needs of everybody else in your life and just put yourself on the list of people you take care of on a regular basis. That's an important skill.

It's also important for people to know that when they're experiencing physical symptoms connected to childhood adversity, it almost always means there are some negative emotions they have repressed. They're not always consciously aware of the presence of those emotions. I want to try to bring them to the surface and I want people to recognize that they are there.

One of the common techniques I'll use is to ask people to imagine their own child experiencing the same adversity they went through, even for just a week. When people think about that, when they do that thought experiment of having their own child or a child that they care about going through that same adversity, it starts to connect them much more accurately with the emotions that are repressed, that are buried, that are being expressed via their bodies.

Once those emotions are brought into a conscious awareness, then we can start talking about them. The patients can start writing about them in a journal or perhaps a letter that won't get mailed, but is written to the Adverse Childhood Experience perpetrators. By converting the bodily expression of emotion into written expression of emotion or spoken expression of emotion, their symptoms start to improve.

Wayne: I've recently been encouraging some of my patients to expressively write about emotions and past traumas. There's been evidence for several decades now of how positive health outcomes come of this type of writing exercise. I think it's a way of expressing yourself on paper to offload built-up negative emotions and thoughts that relate to the physiological manifestation of symptoms.

You mentioned ACE a couple times. The ACE study is a landmark study regarding childhood trauma related to negative health outcomes. This whole concept needs to be addressed in medicine. Would you like to comment on that?

David: Yes, I agree with you, it is a landmark. For me, it's the most important public health study of our generation. It was published by Felitti and Anda as the co-authors, in the American Journal of Preventive Medicine in 1998. It was an enormous study. They took 18,000 people who were coming in for routine checkups, and had them go through a computer-based questionnaire that asked about areas of adversity in childhood. Originally there were seven areas, more recently, it's 10 questions about adversity in childhood.

Then they connected the positive responses to that questionnaire with the health outcomes that occurred to people as adults. They found that about one patient in six had four or more of the adverse childhood experiences. Now, four or more is a really large number, and it's a really significant burden of adversity. That segment of the group suffered enormous negative consequences to their health.

Their incidence of using IV drugs, for example, was 10 times higher than the group that had no ACEs in their background. Alcoholism was five times higher, as was committing domestic violence. Obesity, unexplained physical symptoms, living in poverty, divorce, and multiple sexual partners were also higher. The list just goes on and on.

They also found that it seems childhood adversity activates the body's inflammatory system and can contribute to organ diseases as well, not just psychosocial outcomes. Diabetes, cancer, heart disease, and autoimmune disease were all higher even after you corrected for other risk factors. There was a huge long-term impact. The average age of their population was 51, so these are people who were decades removed from the adversity, and it was still having a negative impact. The summation of all this is that the people with four or more ACEs had a life expectancy 20 years shorter than the people with no ACEs. So it's a huge issue, and very much amenable to intervention. We can help people with these long-term impacts in a way that I'm convinced is going to change their health outcomes.

Wayne: You said in the last 10 years you've committed your career to cause. Obviously, there's massive need in our medical community to bring awareness of these issues so we can help more people. How has the progress been in the past 10 years?

David: Well, it's reaching a tipping point and I think the opioid epidemic is a big part of that. There are 15,000 people per year in the United States alone that die from prescription narcotics. Not illegal narcotics, but ones that are prescribed. The healthcare system is finally taking notice of that, and looking desperately for alternatives.

The psychosocial treatment of stresses that are capable of causing chronic pain and other symptoms is going to be a big part of the future of opioid-free management of chronic pain. People are recognizing that, and there's also a parallel movement toward integrating mental and behavioral health into primary care. The mental and behavioral health professionals that are going to be working alongside doctors in this new system are going to have the expertise to do these stress evaluations that I spoke about earlier, and that's going to make for much better outcomes.

So the information I provide about how to do a stress evaluation and the range of symptoms that can be created through psychosocial stress has become very much in demand. I'm teaching at three different graduate schools, I'm asked to give presentations all over North America and Europe,

I've been involved with three different documentary films about this subject, I'm teaching in an internal medicine residency program. The interest in it is just taking off, and it's been wonderful to see.

Wayne: How can people learn more about you, and this combination of stress and illness?

David: You can certainly start with my book, which is called *They Can't Find Anything Wrong!* You can get information about it through my website, which is stressillness.com. The site has links to other good sources of information as well.

Wayne: I look forward to reading that book soon. Thank you so much for your insights, and your commitment to this bigger cause.

Chapter 6
TIM GEORGE

Tim George is certified by the National Athletic Trainer's Association as an athletic trainer and has worked with athletes of all ages and abilities.

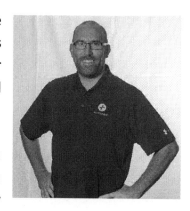

He is the owner and director of an Egoscue Method clinic in San Diego, California, and previously worked at The Egoscue headquarters as a Postural Alignment Specialist. Tim has taught Egoscue Method seminars and workshops to fitness and health care practitioners across the USA and internationally, and has also served as director of the Egoscue Online Therapy Department.

Tim has a bachelor's degree in exercise physiology, and a master's degree in athletic training.

Wayne: Tim George is an exercise therapist who specializes in postural alignment. Welcome, Tim. Let's just go back in time a little bit. Where did you grow up and what was your childhood like?

Tim: I grew up in Lake Forest, California. It's in Orange County, which is in Southern California. Lake Forest was a great place to grow up. I love sports, and was very athletic as a kid, so I played everything under the sun. I had great friends. I just had a great childhood growing up.

I went to El Toro High School. Once you get to a certain age you kind of gravitate towards one sport. Mine was soccer. I played soccer all through high school. Then when I went to college, up in northern California at California State University Chico, I tried playing soccer there. I was a red shirt freshman on the soccer team my first year. But my talents only took me so far, and the next year I didn't make the team.

So I just enjoyed my college time there, and I went into athletic training. My bachelor's degree is in exercise physiology, but my emphasis was always athletic training. With my sports background and love of sports, I thought what better thing to do than get paid to watch people play sports as an athletic trainer. And I've always loved the science in the human body and athletic movement. So it just made sense for me to go into athletic training.

Wayne: So you followed your interest in sports to making a livelihood out of it. What is the best thing about being in this field?

Tim: I really love helping people. So I think it's really that
            time when someone has an "A-ha moment" and they
            really understand what their body is capable of
            doing. I work with people who have debilitating
            lower back pain or hip pain, and they come in saying,
            "Listen, you're my last resort. You're my last hope. I
            don't know what else to do. I've tried everything."
            Then to see that person put in the work, put in the
            dedication, the effort to get their body moving
            correctly and aligned correctly, and you really can
            see how much it impacts and changes their life.
            That's why I got into this, because it's such a great
            thing to be a part of and help someone along that
            journey.

Wayne: So when somebody comes in and their postural
            alignment is less than optimal, what would you say
            are the most common mistakes these patients
            make?

Tim: I don't really look at it as mistakes. When you look at
            someone's postural misalignments, it's a product of
            the world they've created for themselves. A lot of
            clients do think they've made mistakes along the
            way. But we really want clients to understand your
            posture is a product of the world you live in. It's not
            that you did anything wrong. What we want to show
            them and get them to rediscover is that our body
            was designed to be in a certain position, a certain
            alignment. And to no fault of our own, technology

just doesn't require us to move as much as we used to. For that reason, most people sit at a desk on a daily basis. Five, six, seven, eight hours a day.

It doesn't really help our overall health and wellbeing to be sitting this much. So that's where a program like the Egoscue therapy about correcting your posture really becomes something valuable for just about everyone.

Wayne: So lead us into the world of the Egoscue method. What is this therapy?

Tim: Very simply put, it's exercise therapy to correct your posture. That's what we do. And to take that a step further, what we really do at Egoscue is we really help reconnect people to what we believe is the high performance altering vehicle that is the human body. We want to help clients understand that by correcting their posture, they truly can transform their life. We stand by that. We fully believe that.

Because like I said, when people come in to see us, a lot of times they're at their wits end. They've gone through a countless number of well-intentioned health professionals, but they just can't seem to figure out what's causing this pain or how to get themselves out of it. And a lot of times if they can just understand, "Okay, if I can get my body back in better alignment, moving better, it then has the opportunity to heal itself." That's really what the Egoscue method is all about.

Wayne: So when a patient comes in and learns about postural alignment, what is a typical program like for them?

Tim: We'll see most of our clients for a series of visits. The actual number can vary depending on how severe their postural misalignments are, and how bad their symptoms are. But I would say on average we'll see someone anywhere from eight to maybe 10, or up to 16 visits. When clients come in, we'll do an assessment of their postures and we'll take some photos of them from the front, back and the sides. We'll go through their posture with them, and show them the imbalances we're seeing. We'll do some other functional-type tests where we want to really see how their body moves. Give them the posture we're seeing. We'll do a real simple analysis of their gait of how they're walking.

Those functional tests, are really our opportunity to better educate our clients on some of the postural imbalances and the movement imbalances we're seeing. Also, how it ultimately relates back and contributes to the symptoms they came in with. So once we've done that initial evaluation, the functional tests, the gait, and looked at their posture, based on that we'll put together a series of exercises for them. We use a postural analysis software we've developed as a company called EP, which is named after the founder of the company, Peter Egoscue. We'll input their imbalances, their postural analysis into that software. It will suggest some exercises based on what we put in there.

Then as a therapist it's our job then to take our clients through the exercises. And then, make any adjustments we need to make as we get into those exercises. Because, once our clients are doing them, that's where we really start to get a lot of good feedback. We get to really see how much they can and can't do. This really helps us determine what will be the right exercises for them.

Wayne: What about follow up? Is that part of your program?

Tim: It is. Clients are seen a couple times a week for a month to two months. Once they're done with that, it's their job to continue doing the exercises they've learned. And continuing the postural alignment they've been working on while they worked with us. We want to make sure clients understand that we're really trying to build that self-reliance within them, where they really understand the importance of posture to their overall health and wellbeing. And that it's something they need to continue to do forever, from here on out. Because like I said earlier, their posture is a product of the world they've lived in.

And that doesn't change. They're still living in that world. So that's why they need to make sure they understand that posture is something they need to try to maintain and work on a daily basis.

Wayne: So, tell us about a recent patient that you helped. Obviously we don't want to know their name for confidentiality reasons, but talk about their situation and how you helped them.

Tim: Recently a client came in who had been diagnosed with a degenerative hip. MRI's show very little cartilage, pretty close to bone on bone in that hip. Their doctor recommended hip replacement surgery, not immediately, but definitely needed within one to five years. So that person came in with that symptom and that recommendation. Surgery was something they wanted to try to avoid, if not perhaps put off for more than the year to five years that the orthopedic surgeon was recommending.

They've now been with us for about a month. I've seen them a total of four times, on a weekly basis. And their hip pain is probably about 95% better. They're back walking, and moving, and doing some of the activities they like to do. There's still some pain there, but definitely feeling a lot better. And a lot of that contributes to the work they put in to get the body back in alignment and their posture moving in the right direction.

Wayne: Can you explain how a patient with severe hip degeneration seen as bone-on-bone on X-ray, who requires hip replacement surgery, can go through your type of exercises with the Egoscue method, and miraculously find themselves almost pain free? That's amazing!

Tim: The first thing I think everyone needs to understand is that the degeneration of the hip, the bone on bone, the loss of cartilage, is not causing the pain. That's the effect. So the analogy we always use with clients, especially clients that aren't looking to have a hip replacement or a knee replacement, is there's a reason why that hip wore out. There's a reason why that knee wore out. There's a reason why that cartilage is wearing away. You don't want to just replace your car tires without fixing your alignment, right?

What we convey to our clients is the reason that hip wore out. It's not because they're getting old, not because of a family history of bad hips or genetics or anything like that. It wore out because their body is out of alignment. That is something that needs to be corrected. Whether they have the hip replacement or not, that's totally their call, but what we hope to educate our clients on, is we have to get to the cause of why that hip wore out. The bone on bone is not causing pain, because my client is now 95% better, and most of the time is pain free in that hip. That cartilage hasn't regenerated. There's still bone on bone. But their overall position, their overall alignment, their posture has gotten better to where now that hip is able to move the way it was designed to move. That joint is now much better centered. Before, it was out of alignment, which was causing that abnormal wear and tear and that wearing away of the cartilage.

So that's the thing for our clients to understand. The symptom is just that, it's the effect. What we try to do in the Egoscue method is really help our clients understand, let's try to find the cause. Because a lot of times the pain might be in the hip, but the cause might be coming from elsewhere in the body. There might be other misalignments in the body that could be causing or at least contributing to that pain.

Wayne: So this case is severe hip degeneration, wear-in-tear or osteoarthritis. What about other presentations of pain, from headaches to foot pain? Is the same principle applied for these cases?

Tim: Correct. It's still going to be the same. Our mantra is we don't treat symptoms. Our focus is the posture. Our focus is getting the body back in better alignment, working on that postural alignment to really allow the body the opportunity to heal. When our clients come in, we always make sure we say, "Listen, it's not that I don't care about your pain, but where I want us to stay focused is the postural imbalances that are causing that pain. That's what we're going to stay focused on." I think that's one of the unique differences with the Egoscue method. We might be saying it tongue in cheek, but we don't care about the symptom. It doesn't dictate our course of treatment.

What we really focus on is the posture. When we're training new therapists, one of the things we talk to them about is, "Don't get caught up in treating the symptom. Stay focused on the posture. Stay focused on getting the body back in better alignment." So I think that's one of the reasons the Egoscue therapy is so successful. We're not focused on the symptom.

Wayne: As an Egoscue method practitioner, what's the biggest challenge you're facing right now?

Tim: That's a good question. I think for us, it's just letting people know that this is out there. I've been doing this 14 years and I cringe when I hear people say, "This is the best-kept secret out there." I don't want this to be kept a secret. We really want people to know this is an option for them. That's on me as an Egoscue therapist, my staff here, and at all our clinics across the U.S. It's on us to really help spread the word about Egoscue. This is definitely an option for people to look for, in terms of helping get themselves out of pain. So I think right now that's our biggest challenge. How do we reach more people? How do we scale this to where people really come to look at Egoscue. Or they hear the name Egoscue and it becomes common knowledge. Like when someone says yoga, you have an idea of what that is.

We want to get to the point where someone hears Egoscue and immediately thinks, "Yeah, the posture guys. I know that." Our biggest challenge is, how do we reach more people?

Wayne: Is there anything you would like to share that I haven't asked you?

Tim: We've all heard the saying, "You have to see it to believe it." I think with Egoscue and just getting yourself out of pain to begin with, I'd turn it around and say you have to believe it before you see it. Not just with this therapy. But when people are dealing with chronic pain, whatever it might be, I think there just needs to be a belief within themselves that, "I have the right to live pain free. And I believe I can get there. I just have to find the right path, the right journey to get there." I think the clients that have the most success with this therapy are the ones who truly believe they can get better, and are going to continue searching until they find whatever it is that's going to help them get there.

Whether that's Egoscue or something else, I just think there definitely has to be that belief. That's where Pete Egoscue started. He's the founder, and he was the first client of the Egoscue method. He was a Vietnam veteran, a Marine who was shot and wounded. He was doing everything in his power to get better, but just wasn't finding the right path, to getting himself back to feeling pain free. But he always believed he could. He didn't believe this was something he had to live with.

He believed that he could get himself better. He did everything he could, and eventually he said, "You know what, let me see if I can figure this out myself." And he picked up an anatomy book one day and saw that we're designed to be balanced. We're designed to be symmetrical right to left. He didn't look that way. So he decided to try to get there. Which he did. And it all kind of grew from there.

Wayne: Where could people go to learn more about you and this method?

Tim: Go to our website, egoscue.com. It has a lot of good articles, and it has all our clinic locations. We have clinics all over the U.S. People can request more information from the clinic closest to them. Or if they want to learn more, or perhaps try some things on their own, I'd recommend one of Pete Egoscue's books. He's written five of them, all with *Pain Free* in the title. They're on Amazon. The books are a great way to get an introduction to what we do and what the Egoscue method's all about.

Wayne: Thank you Tim, this was very informative. I enjoyed this interview. And I wish you all the best in your endeavors to get people pain free with postural alignment.

Chapter 7
DANA HUMPHREY

Dana Humphrey is the owner and lead publicist at Whitegate PR in Queens, NY, a boutique public relations agency specializing in the pet industry. She also positions herself as a pet expert as "The Pet Lady" and travels coast to coast scouting out the best pet products, brands and pet experts.

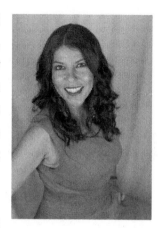

Dana is also a professor and program facilitator at the Fashion Institute of Technology, where she teaches in the pet product marketing and design department.

She was recently named by *Pet Age Magazine* as one of its 40 under 40, and Women of Influence.

Wayne: Dana Humphrey is well known in the pet industry. She owns a public relations firm, and teaches pet product marketing and design at the Fashion Institute of Technology.

But she's here to discuss her personal journey with pain. Dana, many thanks for sharing your story. Let's begin with where you grew up and what your childhood was like.

Dana: It was an international upbringing. I spent six years in London, England, and then spent most of the rest of my life in California. I live in New York now. I was in preschool and kindergarten in England, and then we moved to Northern California, near the San Francisco Bay Area. From there I went to University of San Diego, but I did spend one semester near you, attending Simon Fraser University in Burnaby, British Columbia.

I think I spent most of my childhood a little bit as a loner. I was usually found in the library finding some books to read or out playing with the boys, playing soccer.

Wayne: When did this pain experience start for you?

Dana: I have some notes from teachers along the way on my report cards, that I've always been a daydreamer, and I've always been spending time drifting off. I think I spent a lot of my childhood very uncomfortable. But the specific time that I can recall the pain really setting in, was actually about 10 months ago.

Wayne: Do you know what triggered the pain to come on?

Dana: A lot of things were happening at the same time. I was working a lot and traveling a lot for work, flying from New York City to Florida for a trade show where I had a lot going on. Then my grandmother passed away while I was there. I was also going through some changes in my relationship. It was just a lot of things stewing at once. I woke up with this excruciating pain in my top left shoulder, and basically spent the next couple of days agonizing over it. I had also run a 10K race, which at the time I thought exacerbated it.

But I was never really sure about the source. A lot of people were trying to tell me that it could be physical. I had been at a wedding and been dancing, and I had been skiing, and then I was on a boat, so there were always a lot of variables in my life. Finally, after a few months of soul-searching and being in a lot of pain, I picked up a book by Dr. John Sarno called *Healing Back Pain: The Mind-Body Connection*, and that was a game changer for me.

I had spent a couple of weeks lying on the couch, not able to sleep because I was in so much pain. I was trying everything. I was going to the chiropractor. I was going to acupuncture. I was trying lots of different types of pain medication, and nothing really seemed to be helping. When I was sitting in my acupuncturist's office, I saw that book, picked it up, and couldn't put it down. I got through to chapter three while I was still in the waiting room.

In the book, Dr. Sarno was explaining about a "type T" personality, which is almost like a type A, but increased. And it seemed to fit my lifestyle perfectly as far as being really extreme in everything I do, and having really high expectations. I realized that the pain I was experiencing was most likely trapped emotions in my body.

I picked up the book on a Friday. By Sunday, my pain was completely gone.

Wayne: That's a remarkable turnaround from 10 months of pain. Your experience, trying many different specialties and therapies, doctor visits, medications, is a very common story for patients with chronic pain. That's certainly what I find in my practice. That book is a phenomenal read for anyone interested in learning the basics of how chronic pain is a mind-body condition. That's when the mind directly influences the body and acts as one.

Dr. Sarno was an amazing pioneer in this field of mind-body medicine and has inspired many people to take on this different approach. How has it been for you?

Dana: It's funny, when I told this story to a good friend of mine, she said, "It's like you're experiencing cognitive mind-body for the first time." Maybe I was. It seemed to all click. I know that I have repressed emotions. That's something I guess I didn't want to look at. I didn't want to see it. But since reading the book, I've really been able to shift my perspective about how I experience pain, and it's really helped me.

One important thing he says in the book is that only about five percent of people are able to really handle this concept. I've been on a spiritual conscious path for the past couple years, so after trying everything and spending a lot of money on different treatments, I really believe a lot of the things I was doing were working, because I believed in them, and they had a placebo effect.

Acupuncture was working, because I thought it was working. So I would go for a treatment, and I would feel a little better. Or I'd go to the chiropractor, and I'd feel better for a few hours. Understanding that my mind played a big role in that, and understanding the importance of the placebo effect, was really a game changer.

That first weekend when I picked up the book, I had planned actually a big bike ride for that Saturday. It was going to be a 25-mile ride to the beach with some friends, then a 25-mile ride home, a total of 50 miles. Pre-back pain I had done things like that all the time. But now I was a little scared, and I wasn't sure how I was going to do.

This was in May. Remember, I live in New York City, and after a cold winter you want to be outside when the weather turns nice. In the book, Dr. Sarno said to maintain your physical activities and keep going. Don't be scared to do things, because the pain isn't from something physical, so doing something physical can't make it worse.

I wasn't fully on board with that concept. But I realized I could do the bike ride one of two ways. I could be in fear, just thinking, "Let's go slow. Take it easy," being afraid of everything coming my way. Or, I could go into the bike ride just trying to embrace it for all it is. That attitude really helped me. By proving to myself I could do this bike ride and not be in pain, or be in the same amount of pain whether I was sitting on the couch or on the bike, really helped me get out there and feel good and have fun.

And by doing it, you benefit from all of the good things of going for a bike ride, that stimulate your body. I had spent a month or two not being physical, which added to my not feeling well. So that was really important, just reading that and understanding, "Okay, there's something bigger here. I probably have some repressed emotions in my body. I think that's probably true. Actually I know that's true."

It's not something I'm really gung-ho about looking into, but if that's going to help me, I'll do it, and it's free. I'm not having to go to all these different treatments that are costing thousands of dollars.

Wayne: In Dr. Sarno's book, he talks about many patients whose other ailments or conditions disappear or drastically improve with this approach of mind-body awareness. Have you had any personal experience of this? Have you been able to share your story to help others?

Dana: Yes. Now I have a whole different perspective about pain in general. There are people in my life who have pain. I think I've been able to be helpful to them in as gentle a way as possible, trying to help them look at the fact that maybe it's not something physical.

Also for me, the pain actually started in my left hip a few years ago. I now believe that it moved up to my left shoulder. Now it's actually moved to my right shoulder. But I have a different perspective when it comes on.

I said it was gone completely, and it was for a while. This past fall it came back a little bit, and I had my original reaction as soon as it was coming on. I went for a road trip, and I had this fear that because I was driving, somehow the physical part of sitting in a car and driving would bring on the pain. And so it did. I immediately went to my same old solutions of, "Okay, I need an Advil," all these needs that I have of go-to pain solutions.

Over the next couple days, the pain was getting a lot worse because I was adding my own fear and anxiety to it. But then I remembered what I had read. I went to a Zen Buddhist meditation, and was reminded that adding the judgment of the pain is what's making me suffer. So the pain's there. Sure, I can feel it coming on. It's just a sensation. But if I add to it all this baggage of, "Oh my God, it's back. What am I going to do?" All this fear and bad self-talk, it makes it a bigger problem.

Since then, it went down again. Now the past couple of weeks I feel it again in my top right shoulder, but I'm not letting it run my life. I'm not letting it debilitate me in the way I had before. I haven't taken any pain medication. I'm letting it be there. I shifted my attitude to how I feel about the pain. The low level of pain that's there, can be there for as long as it needs to, because that's just my new attitude about it, so it makes it not as bad.

Wayne: Excellent. Thank you so much for sharing your journey and how it's been an internal one, to really deal with pain and master pain, so you can actually live your life. You can do your activities. You can do your meditation, and have a more enjoyable life. Not only that, but you can also help other people on the journey, which is fantastic. Your story is inspiring.

Where can people learn more about you?

Dana: They can find more about me at our website www.whitegatepr.com/about-us/.

Chapter 8
NAMAN KUMAR

Naman Kumar is the Founder and CEO of Airo Health in Waterloo, Ontario. The company is committed to inventing health technology that helps people to not worry about their health, and feel good about themselves.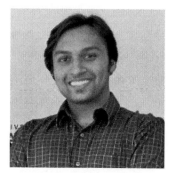

Airo is the developer of *Airo for Stress*, a wristband and app that serve as a 24/7 assistant, helping people build mental strength. The technology tracks people's anxiety and recommends stress-reducing tweaks to their daily routine.

Wayne: Naman Kumar has a very special technique of helping people with pain, called Neurofeedback. Naman, thank you for sharing your story. Let's begin by going back in time. Where did you grow up, and what was your childhood like?

Naman: It's an interesting story. At this point in time, I've spent about half my life in India and half in Canada. I was born in Delhi, India, moved to Canada at 13, and I've been here ever since. I graduated from high school in Fort McMurray and then ended up at the University of Waterloo studying engineering.

But growing up I had a huge interest in both biology and engineering. I couldn't decide what to do. So when I was studying engineering, I kept up with the advances in biology as much as I could. My main interest was the cardiovascular system and the nervous system - their regular functioning, and how they interact with each other. It's just super-fascinating.

Wayne: How did you end up combining biology and engineering in a career?

Naman: I think life is about growth, which means you're constantly learning, and each day you're challenging yourself with something you didn't know before. For me, having that life means operating a startup. It's about building something from nothing by bringing together knowledge, not only from engineering and biology, but also human behaviour.

My startup is called Airo Health. It's based on engineering principles that are used to help people.

Wayne: So you're mingling the two disciplines of biology and engineering and coming up with actual solutions for health based on science.

Naman: Yes, that's exactly what we're doing.

Wayne: Please describe how Neurofeedback works to achieve health and pain reduction.

Naman: Fundamentally, Neurofeedback is about working with sympathetic and parasympathetic parts of the nervous system. The sympathetic component involves the "fight or flight" response. It's stimulated when you find yourself in a stressful situation, like running into a brown bear when you're out for a jog in the woods, or when you're getting agitated about deadlines. The stressful event triggers the sympathetic response, which causes the subconscious mind and nervous system to work in conjunction to pump adrenaline, which in turn stimulates the heart to increase its cardiac output. The extra blood flow to the muscles helps you fight the situation or flee from it. The whole body is under siege and the response is to survive.

The parasympathetic component is involved in the polar opposite. That's the "relaxation response" which causes reduced heart rate, reduced blood pressure, reduced oxygen supply to the muscles, and generally whole-body relaxation. Two examples of this are after you have a big dinner and feel relaxed, or are sitting quietly and mediating.

In our day-to-day activities there are constant fluctuations between the stress response and relaxation response, with the sympathetic and parasympathetic nervous systems controlling our hormones, neuropeptides and neurotransmitters.

We want to make sure our bodies maintain their normal rhythm of sympathetic and parasympathetic activity. But if you're under continuous stress, the sympathetic component takes over. Now it dominates, and doesn't let the parasympathetic response activate. That's when Airo Health can step in with our device that ties to your wrist like a Fitbit, but for stress, anxiety and pain. It will literally track your nervous system every second of every day and as soon as it starts to detect that the sympathetic response, or "fight or flight" state is becoming more dominant, it will beep ever so slightly. Which is a sign to you. It's like telling yourself, "I'm getting stressed, I should do something to change it".

The sooner you do something about that stress, the better. It prevents you from spiraling down into the negative parts of stress with anxiety and pain.

Wayne: Excellent. Thank you for that explanation. So people can buy your Airo device to put on their wrist to monitor their stress response in the day. When they get the warning, could they stop their activity and take a minute to do breathing exercises, and stimulate their relaxation response via the parasympathetic nervous system?

Naman: That's right. A huge amount of research shows that when you are stressed, the number one thing you need to do is acknowledge it. From there you can change it.

What the Airo does, is vibrate and send a signal to the mobile app on your smart phone. The app will show you a notification as soon as you click it. It will take you to a small journal where you can quickly jot down what's going on with you right now. Making that note is important so you can know what actually caused that stress.

Then, once you've acknowledged it and you want to change it, we suggest a breathing exercise called "resonant breathing". It's a special personalized breathing exercise where you breathe at the rate where you feel calm. You will become relaxed within 30-60 seconds. That's how it works.

This is not something we invented. It's been known to medical science for a very long time now. But now, mobile technology and mobile devices can bring people moment-by-moment information that enhances their health.

Wayne: At medical school or studying science at University, you learn how the brain communicates with the body via the nervous system, endocrine system and circulatory system. It's wonderful to take these principles and use technology to identify instant changes in the nervous system in real time with people's lives. Within a minute of resonant breathing exercise, they can literally start to see changes in their physiology and thus their stress levels coming down. We know when stress levels come down, we can heal, we can improve, and we can have less anxiety, less depression and less pain. We get a multitude of health benefits when we're aware, proactive and actually start controlling it all.

Is there anything else you'd like to share about Neurofeedback?

Naman: I would say it's an objective measurement of how your body's doing at one point in time. Neurofeedback measures heart rate variability. It's a tangible way to measure what's going on with your body. All of us would benefit from knowing how our own stress response works. Maybe we are stressed all the time or sometimes only at specific moments in the day. But you don't have to guess what's going on. You just look at the number on the mobile app and start resonant breathing to bring a relaxation response into your life moment by moment. Think of a car traveling 50 miles per hour when the speed limit is 30. We see the number on our speedometer, and adjust our speed. This is the same way. We can glance at the number and make adjustments for optimal health. We should all take advantage of that as soon as possible.

Wayne: These are good insights. I really appreciate the focus on objective measurements, as we in medicine rely on them to optimize our assessments. It's extremely difficult to assess pain accurately, as it's a subjective experience. So when you can move into a realm of measuring the body's response to pain, stress and anxiety through heart rate variability, we have the ability to self-treat conditions often unsuccessfully treated with traditional methods.

For those wondering, heart rate variability is the variable waveform between each beat of the heart. Science has used it for decades to measure stress responses. Researchers at HeartMath Institute in California are showing positive health outcomes with heart-based meditations. There's an informative book about that called *The HeartMath Solution* by Doc Childre and Howard Martin.

What you're doing with Airo can help us measure and treat with resonant breathing exercises to control our heart variability and stress response, and more toward a greater health experience and less pain. I think this is a leading-edge approach, which can easily be incorporated on a large scale when more people are aware of it. So how can people learn more about the product, and about you?

Naman: We have much more information at AiroHealth.com. The website has a number of scientific studies that talk about the science and technology. There's more information about me there as well.

Wayne: Naman, thanks for joining me and sharing this information.

Chapter 9

JOSEPH LACKIE

Joseph Lackie is the president of Bud & Herbs LTD, a medical cannabis company in Vancouver, British Columbia.

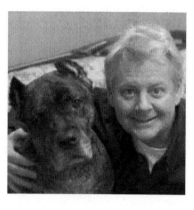

Bud & Herbs offers online and in-store distribution of medical marijuana, along with training, continuing education, and certification for dispensary agents and staff, along with resellers. The company also offers Hemp-based Neutraceutical CBD products.

Previously Joe founded two other companies in the technology sector.

Wayne: Joe Lackie is a longtime student of the cannabis industry and the founder of a medicinal marijuana company. He also has a personal connection to this, having mastered chronic pain through medical cannabis. Joe, thank you for sharing your story. Let's begin with your younger years and your experience with pain.

Joe: I grew up in Kelowna, British Columbia. I had a troubled youth. I started out in professional motocross for 12 years and won a couple provincial championships. The downside of that of course, was I had many crashes with many concussions and there's probably not a part of my body that hasn't been beaten by that sport. Then once I got out of motocross, I went back and played rugby. I played third division rugby for the Calgary Hornets. I played for another 10 years till I went into the refereeing end of it just because of the pain. Then I retired from refereeing in 2005. My knees just couldn't take it anymore.

Wayne: What type of business were you involved in before the marijuana industry?

Joe: I was in the tech industry. I was the founder of Titan Integrated Technology, an IT company here in Vancouver. Our focus was mainly the film industry. Over 17 years we've done over 450 productions and did a lot of data security design for them. I was also the founder of a company called Shieldcore, which was a UNIX based data security appliance that we went global with. In 2012, I went through some ailments and sold the company, and then my focus was on medical cannabis to treat all the symptoms I have.

Wayne: How did you originally stumble across marijuana as a treatment?

Joe: I was in Hawaii with a bunch of guys, with motocross and skateboarding. We were sitting down one day and they were passing around a Hawaiian marijuana joint. The gentleman I was with grabbed my hand and said, "No, no, no, bro. That's not the one for you, try this one." That was the one he used himself for pain management. There was no "stone" out of it. When you took a drag, you could feel just the pain going away from your body but you wouldn't get stoned.

I was totally intrigued with it. It was a very seedy cannabis, so when I got back to Canada, of course I took the seeds and grew that plant, and that was the product I used for all the years. So that's how I got into it.

Wayne: Now many years later, and you have this vast knowledge of cannabis. Tell us a little bit about the journey to where you are now.

Joe: Well, I was very blessed with the technology industry. I learned a lot about correlation. Unfortunately in North America I couldn't find any information, which is sad. But once I started looking on the internet using the technology we had, I found tremendous resources through Europe. Countries like Germany and Sweden, with university studies. So I studied everything and became a student of the industry. I took as much knowledge as I could and I developed all our products. The information is out there, you just have to know how to find it. That's what I did. I studied all the universities. The studies from Helsinki, and the other major universities. I took that information and developed my own products from that.

It was a lot of trial and error. Because the big thing is, when I first started, CO_2 extraction wasn't available. It was mainly done with different solvents. The evolution to where we are today has been quite the journey. But I just thank the Good Lord that he's provided me with all that information and we're able to help people and also myself. I'm not a big fan of narcotics at all. When I had my tech companies, I had to have the clearest head and unfortunately it was still reefer madness, so I couldn't tell people I was on a very high CBD strain, because they just didn't understand. That's how I got to where I am today. Again, it's all through learning, knowledge and just trying to source everything.

Wayne: Can you just share what are the basic properties of marijuana that help people's pain?

Joe: Marijuana is broken down into different parts. Basically the two we're mainly concerned with are

THC, the Tetrahydrocannabinol and CBD, the Cannabidiol. There are also CBGs and CBNs, and we also do a lot with terpenes, but we don't need to talk about those. The two main ones we focus on are the THC and the CBD.

Wayne: When you talk about these products, is there a ratio you find ideal for chronic pain?

Joe: The ratio depends on the person. Everybody is different. Everybody reacts differently to it. We always start people off on Cannabidiol, CBDs. The reason for that is, people are still scared of getting high. And we don't want to get them high. I've also learned that CBD is a wonderful substance. Probably 80% of the time, once people use the CBDs, if it's great, we stop there. There's no use going any farther with them by throwing the THC in.

Now, with the more excruciating pain, we bring the THC into it. One thing I've learned is, I'm a very big fan of small doses. To see how the people react to it. If we need to increase the dose, of course we can do that. What we've found that is working the best for us right now, with basic pain levels, is what we call a one-to-one ratio. For instance, one of our products contains 7.5 milligrams of CBD and 7.5 milligrams of THC. Our research has shown us by having those equal numbers, you get the benefits of the CBD working with the Cannabidiol system. But also, the THC helps the inflammation.

But also what goes on with the two is CBD counter-reacts the psychoactive effects of THC. So people get unbelievable pain relief with maybe just a touch of euphoria. Again, depending on the extremities of the injuries, whether we're treating cancer or just regular pain, that's the basis I use. Start at a very low dose, and then work with them and the physicians of course, to find the dosing that works best for them. That's really the secret, working with the doctors and listening to the patients, and just doing your very best to find the optimal dose for them.

Of course there are also different delivery methods, which is very important when you're talking to the patients. What they're comfortable with. We deal with a lot of seniors, and we find with them, the chew tablet is best. It's easy for them to ingest and it just works the best for them.

Wayne: Thank you for the insights. We have a quagmire of a situation for us doctors, because we know it can help some patients but we're also concerned about its purity and adverse side effects. As a doctor prescribing medication, you really need to know and trust what you are prescribing for your patients. How pure are your products and how do you achieve that level of purity?

Joe: It's been an evolution of development. First, we start with the very best organic flower you can get. It's very important that there are no herbicides or pesticides in that. Because of course when you concentrate a product that has herbicides and pesticides, that concentration goes into the product and is very bad for patients.

What we do is, we take that organic cannabis flower and we extract the CO_2 from it, then we use a proprietary distillation process to remove all the waxes and plant matter. Once they're gone, that's how we get into the 99.6, 99.7% purity. Then we do a content analysis. Everything is tested and it gives us all the results.

After that we take our product and get it third-party tested, to make sure it has the confirmed best purity out there. That's the key moving forward with everything. Unfortunately, not a lot of people do that, but we're trying to set the bar to excellence.

Wayne: You've actually won some awards for your products. Tell us about that.

Joe: There is something called the *Tokers Bowl*. It is the most prestigious competition out there. It was never hosted by any of the nutrient companies. I have the first place trophy right here. We grew it under the name "the unknown grower" because I couldn't let people know what I was doing. We called the product *Lizard* because we had a Savannah monitor that would cruise around our plants and eat all the bugs. But the big thing is, we do have the very best product in the world and I have the trophy to prove it.

Wayne: What are the cost of your products?

Joe: We try to give clients the very best value we can. The costs are coming down considerably because of the extraction processes. The average cost out there is based on the amount of THC in the product. In the marketplace today, a good number is $12 per hundred milligrams of pure THC. That's what the prices are based on now. Unfortunately, there are some unscrupulous people who say they have that number, but when we test it, it's not close. We test a lot of the products we find, just to keep them honest. And it's just embarrassing what they're doing.

Wayne: You mentioned clinical studies in the past. Where are you at with that process?

Joe: Currently we're in the process of clinical studies in Eastern Canada. One of the studies we're doing now is looking at diabetic pain. They've had the first five patients in it. Of course until we have documentation, I can't go into the details because in this industry it has to be exact facts and exact studies. But as soon as they're made public, we'll be able to share them.

In addition to the diabetic pain, we're also working with a Toronto based pain clinic for many pain conditions. We hope to publish the papers soon. I'm looking forward to sharing the documentation. Because I'm all about education and sharing, and that's how we're really going to win the battle of the cannabis wars.

Wayne: What is your biggest challenge right now?

Joe: The biggest challenge right now is the bad information that's out there. It's really sad. I call it "fake experts". There are people who have a PhD from my industry or the technology industry, they go online for a couple of hours and study what's going on. These are the people that are hired as speakers. When I listen to some of the stuff they say, I get angry because they're giving the wrong information to people, which is really hurting our industry. It really is. So the challenge is getting the correct information out there.

Wayne: Is there something you'd like to share that we haven't already discussed?

Joe: One of the big things I see happening, and I hear people talking about, especially in North America, is everyone needs money for research. "We have to start the research." But the research is already out there. You have to go and get it, like I did. And doing a global collaboration with the universities. Right now, Canada is five years behind. The biggest thing is we need to welcome the research that has been done globally to advance it to the next level.

Wayne: Can you share some information about where people can go to learn more about your products and what we've been talking about today?

Joe: The best source right now is the website, budsgeneralstore.com. We have all the information on every product and the links to the university studies we used to create them. Plus, I'm doing a video on each of the products to try to answer anyone's questions. Because the most important thing right now is to give patients or members as much information as possible, to make the right decision. I can't prescribe any medication, but we're very blessed that there are a lot of doctors who are now recognizing it. So it's important to share the information with them to get the best treatments for their patients.

Wayne: Joe, thank you so much for enlightening us about medical cannabis. It's a subject more and more people will want to know about.

Chapter 10
JAMES MCCORMACK

Dr. James McCormack holds a doctorate in pharmacy. He is a professor on the Faculty of Pharmaceutical Sciences at the University of British Columbia, Vancouver Campus.

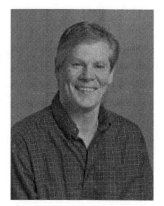

Dr. McCormack has extensive experience, both locally and internationally, talking to health professionals and consumers about the rational use of medication, and has presented more than 300 seminars on drug therapy. His focus is shared-informed decision-making, using evidence-based information and rational therapeutic principles.

He has also published more than 100 articles, mainly in the area of rational drug therapy, and has been an editor for two internationally-recognized textbooks on appropriate/rational drug therapy.

Wayne: Dr. James McCormack is a professor of pharmaceutical sciences at the University of British Columbia, and cohost of the widely acclaimed Best Science Medicine podcast that's been running for 10 years here in Canada. Thank you so much, James, for joining me.

Let's go back in time. Where did you grow up and go to university?

James: I was actually born in England, and when I was a young child in the mid-60s my family emigrated to Canada. Most of my training has been at the University of British Columbia, but I received my doctorate at the Medical University of South Carolina. I've been here at UBC since the 80s, teaching and helping people try to understand medical evidence. What we know about medications, how to think about them and how to use them. I do this because when you look critically at how medications are used, I'm sure everyone will be "shocked", but they're not used perfectly. So we try to talk about how to look at evidence, how to look at studies and how to put it all into clinical context. We primarily do this for healthcare providers because they're the ones that are using most of the prescription medications. But we also do it with patients because ultimately they're the people who take the medications. So it's all about knowledge dissemination and helping people understand the information.

Wayne: So let's talk about chronic pain medications, the evidence behind using them and the effectiveness of these drugs.

James: When we're talking about chronic pain a lot of the discussion has to come down to how we think about using medications. I just talked about evidence. There's a thing called evidence-based practice. That's when your healthcare provider works with patients and uses the best available evidence and their clinical expertise or experience, and then patients' values and preferences. When it comes to chronic pain, there are a variety of different ways of evaluating whether or not a particular pain medication works in a study. So we can say these drugs seem to have an effect when we look at the average person in a study, but that doesn't mean in any way, shape or form it's going to work in everybody. And it may or may not work in an individual patient. That's where shared decision-making and individual assessment comes in.

Unfortunately, when it comes to things like chronic pain, when you assess many pain medications in studies to see whether they're effective, in general they don't produce a large benefit. For years and years we've used medications like acetaminophen or Tylenol, and the evidence is exceedingly weak that it actually works much better than placebo. The way we test to see whether something works for pain is to take a bunch of people that have, for example, osteoarthritis pain or neuropathic pain or back pain, and then randomize them to take either acetaminophen or a placebo three or four times a day for a number of weeks. Then we look to see if there's any difference in the amount of pain they're having. Interestingly, when it comes to something like acetaminophen, a very commonly used pain medication, it doesn't seem to work that much better than a placebo.

So even though acetaminophen is often used as the first thing we use early on in the treatment of chronic pain, the evidence is reasonably clear that it doesn't do a whole heck of a lot. So that's sort of where we're starting from with regard to the evidence. But, some people will report it works well for them. So that's where it kind of gets tricky. A typical study would compare acetaminophen to placebo and what we typically might find is, and I'm just going to give some ballpark numbers, you might get about 30% of people in the placebo group reporting that they are feeling less pain. This is despite the fact you haven't really given them anything. Whereas in the people who actually got acetaminophen, instead of 30%, you might get 35% or 40% reporting a benefit. So it does have some effect, but most people aren't benefitting. And in fact in some studies – for instance back pain -

acetaminophen doesn't show any greater benefit than placebo.

So as a healthcare provider, if I was to recommend acetaminophen for your chronic pain, about 30% of you would come back and say, "I think that worked reasonably well." The problem is, it wasn't because of the medication. It was either the placebo effect, which is probably of some benefit in people with chronic pain, but it's likely just the natural fluctuation of chronic pain. All of that is very difficult to tease out. And even if someone thinks they've benefitted, one of the most important things to do is re-evaluate by either lowering the dose or stopping the medication on a semi-regular basis to see if it is really doing anything.

The same thing applies to medications like aspirin or ibuprofen. Those medications are called NSAIDS. The studies for those show a little bit more benefit for some conditions than acetaminophen, especially for things like osteoarthritis pain. But again, all we can do is offer advice and say try them and see if they work for you. Start with a low dose, and if you get benefit, great, and if you don't, that's unfortunate. That's sort of the general approach to using over the counter medications. There are a lot of other medications, obviously narcotics or opioids and other agents like some antidepressants that have an effect on chronic pain. There is some evidence that they are better than placebo, but again, most people don't get a benefit from these treatments.

Wayne: Thank you for introducing that principle of using acetaminophen and nonsteroidal anti-inflammatories. Let's move on. A family physician will see many patients with neuropathic pain that may be coming from the nerve roots exiting the spine being impinged by herniated disks or overgrowths of bone called osteophytes, or alternatively from tight painful muscles surrounding the spine that are causing burning, shooting or electric-type pain. As general practitioners, we spend most of our time treating chronic pain by prescribing different types of medications like amitriptyline, cymbalta or the infamous narcotics. Let's dive in and talk about the evidence for these regularly-prescribed medications.

James: I work with a group in Alberta that's a very evidence-based group of family doctors and physicians. We recently looked at much of the evidence around treatments for neuropathic pain. A number of the medications you mentioned have been studied. For example, amitriptyline is a very old antidepressant we've used for many years. As I was talking about with medications like acetaminophen and the NSAIDS, the way we study these things is we randomize people with neuropathic pain to either amitriptyline/duloxetine/gabapentin or placebo and we look to see, over a period of weeks or so, how many people are feeling better. By feeling better, what we typically use as an endpoint is a 30% reduction in pain scores. That's what we consider an effective treatment. The results vary, but we see anywhere from about one in four to about one in ten people getting a benefit above placebo. What I'm trying to say is not everybody, by any stretch of the imagination, gets a benefit. Some of the more effective ones are some of the older medications. With medications like amitriptyline about one in four people will get a clinically important benefit, but that means three out of four don't.

That's why it's so important that when a healthcare provider makes these recommendations, we say we're hoping this might provide some benefit, but it likely won't have much of an effect. I'm not being a great salesman here, but we're talking about the reality of what we see with these agents. Now, just as I said with other medications, in the placebo group a number of people do report getting better. So that's why it is always important to try to figure out when someone does get better, is it the medication or just the natural pain fluctuation. Roughly speaking, about 50 percent of people who get a medication will appear to get a benefit, but about half if not more of those people are not getting benefit because of the medication. So it gets very, very tricky.

Wayne: Okay, so looking at a medication like amitriptyline. You're saying 25% are going to get better from the drug and about 25-30% are going to get better from the fact that they're just taking a drug that the doctor believes is good. Therefore, there's a 25-30% response to placebo.

James: Right. So if that's the case we need to do constant re-evaluation and say, "Let's actually stop the medication and see if your pain comes back, because that's probably the best way to figure out if it's actually working for you." I think for most people, once you've got pain control you don't want to play around with it, but if people were aware it's unlikely that it was the medication helping, it's worth giving it a trial to just stop it because all these medications have side effects. Now most people don't get these side effects, but because many of these medications have what we call central nervous system effects, they affect a whole bunch of receptors and a number of people will get things like dry mouth or sedation or dizziness or nausea and that sort of stuff. It's all about finding the balance of the benefit and the harm.

Ultimately, a healthcare provider cannot in any way, shape or form tell you the right dose for you. But one of the best ways to reduce the chance of side effects from these medications is to start with very, very low doses and work your way up. Because some of these medications do have some long-term side effects. Some of the antidepressants are difficult to get off because you can go through withdrawal. We all know about the problem with opioids and becoming physically dependent on those medications. It's all about choosing medications for which we have reasonably good evidence with an understanding of the harms, and allowing the person to try to figure out if it works and what is the correct dose. No treatment for chronic pain is successful in 100% of people. It's all about trial and error.

Wayne: It's interesting you mentioned lower doses. In the past, I've seen patients who had seen specialists who are genuinely trying to help their patient by starting a low dose of medication and then titrate up to five times higher than the initial dose. I just think, "Oh my goodness, what are the side effects and how will this impact their lives in the future?" It amazes me that low doses can be just as good, if not better, than higher doses.

James: It's tricky. This actually applies to almost all medications. You get most of the effect of a medication from a quarter of the dose. Now, will there be a small percentage of people who get better with higher doses? Absolutely. Can any healthcare provider figure that out? No. The only person who can figure that out is the patient, and so the best way to try and figure this out is to let the person know that most of these medications will have an effect on something like neuropathic pain within a few days. You don't need to use these medications for months and months to figure out if they're going to work. So you can use a very low dose to start and see if you get a bit of a benefit. If you think you might be getting a bit of a benefit and no side effects, that's great.

You could try doubling the dose, and see what happens, but realizing as soon as you start increasing the dose you're at a greater risk of having these side effects I mentioned, whether it be dizziness or dry mouth or nausea or whatever. Many people will tolerate or get tolerance to those sort of side effects, but our job is to try to make you feel better, not make you feel worse with medications. When a good majority of people who we give medications don't get benefit from them, we need to work with an understanding of that concept. It's nothing to be embarrassed about, it is just the reality of the situation. You shouldn't feel bad if your doctor gives you a pain medication and it doesn't work. You just need to say, "It didn't seem to work." We have a sort of funny byline we use with our evidence-based group. It's, "We don't care". When we say that, what we mean is we don't care if you take medications or not. We do care that the medications you're on are working for you. We're not going to take it personally if that medication isn't working.

It's our job to help you find that right medication. With chronic pain, it would be quite unusual for any medication to get rid of it all, so the expectation is we want to be able to manage it. What we don't want is to have you on four or five different medications that then interact with each other, and then you get side effects from all of them, and then we end up overall making things worse. So, it's a bit of a game that you have to play. And to play the game you need to know the rules. And the rules are, as healthcare providers all we can do is provide some guidance. We cannot definitively say, "This is going to work better than that," because often there are no studies that actually compare these agents for us to give you this type of any advice. It's really got to be done individually. In fact, that applies to every medication we've ever had, whether it be for pain or any other condition. It's all about individualizing the dose and being careful not to cause side effects.

Wayne: That's certainly something I find with patients. There are occasional miraculous results. Several patients come to mind where the pain virtually vanished, but it's only a handful of people who get those amazing outcomes. For most patients the pain medication will have no effect or just a slight reduction in pain. Often patients go through a cycle of medication trial and error until you find either the best drug or combination of drugs.

James: Yes, it's really important to appreciate this concept. From personal experience, over the last several years I had some sort of back pain or hip pain, which I had looked at and assessed. I never tried any pain medications because I don't really believe they all have a great effect. I wanted to find the cause of it. Often for back pain you can do injections of steroids into sites to see if you can improve the outcome. Nothing seemed to work, but then after about two and a half years I had this one injection. At the time it didn't seem to work, but then two weeks later my pain was gone. Now, I have no idea whether it was that injection. It could have been, but the pain could have just gone away. That's the interesting thing about these things and it's why you need constant re-evaluation. The thing is, I actually don't care how it went away. I'm just glad it did. I got lucky.

The issue is even if a person comes back and says, "Boy, it's way better," it could have just been that it got better. Now, much of chronic pain obviously doesn't disappear, and clearly it's not going to miraculously get better for people who are in severe pain from cancer and so on. We do need to use medications properly to control that, but it's really important to always re-evaluate. As a healthcare provider we should say, "I'm thrilled your pain is better because that's what we were trying to do. Why don't we see if the benefit was because of the treatment or if it just got better on its own." Like I said, the best way to do that is to take a person who has effective pain relief and then start whittling back on their medications and seeing if changing the dose has any effect. We can always restart the medication if the pain gets worse. I'm not aware of any evidence that says if you stop the medication and the pain comes back then you can't get it under control again. I've heard people say that's an issue, but certainly for neuropathic pain that really doesn't make much sense at all. So that's basically the approach. Again, it's an individualized approach, and it's what we should be doing every day in medicine.

Wayne: Can you inform our readers about the new website that looks at the evidence for different types of pain medications with percentages for the placebo effect and drug effectiveness?

James: Interestingly enough, a lot of healthcare providers really don't have a good grasp on how to look at evidence. This is not a criticism. It's a tricky thing to do, especially when it comes to looking at the evidence around pain medications. There are many, many studies. What we want to do is try to help healthcare providers and patients figure out what drug to try first and then second etc. As I said before, the group I work with in Alberta put in a lot of work looking at all the best available evidence they could find for neuropathic pain. There are around five different types of medication treatments that seem to have some reasonable evidence that they can have an effect on neuropathic pain.

We created a website at pain-calculator.com. It's a calculator where you can click on the different treatments, and it will give you information about how effective a potential medication could be. But realizing that, again, in you specifically we don't know if it's going to be effective. However, at least we can give you a good idea about the evidence for its effectiveness, and also list the side effects you might experience, and how big of a benefit, and the costs. All these medications have costs associated with them. But there's none that really stand out above any other one. Typically, you should start with the least expensive of these because there's nothing to guide a person to say this is one is on average that much better or this one is that much better tolerated. We hope this information just helps the discussion you can have with your healthcare provider about what benefit might be expected, and the harms and the costs.

Wayne: Thank you for that. One final question, is there something you'd like to share that we haven't already discussed?

James: I really think it's so important to empower patients to understand that the decisions are ultimately theirs. It's the patient who ends up taking the medication, not the health care provider. So it's all about what we call shared decision-making. To do shared decision-making you have to know the best available evidence. You have to be with a healthcare provider who has some good clinical experience and can help you work your way through this, but ultimately it's your values and preferences that are going to help you make that decision. It's all about you and your healthcare provider maneuvering through the minefield, if you will, of medications. There are some really useful medications that can have an effect on pain, but like I said, they benefit at most, one in four people. When you look at things like the cannabinoids or medical marijuana for neuropathic pain we're talking only about one in eight, maybe one in ten getting a benefit. Now it's great that one in eight or one in ten get a benefit, but medical marijuana can also have side effects, just like the high-dose opioids or the antidepressants or the other pain medications that we use for neuropathic pain.

There's nothing magical about this. It's working with that healthcare provider with the best evidence, their expertise and getting feedback from you to help them help you as best they can.

Wayne: Absolutely I agree with that. It's all about having a good conversation with patients and understanding their needs and wants and coming up with choices together. I think without the evidence it's impossible to do that, but with the evidence, the facts and figures you're mentioning, then at least we're going forward, giving the best care we can with pharmaceuticals and their management. Thank you so much, James. I really appreciate you sharing your insights.

Chapter 11
CINDY PERLIN

Cindy Perlin is the author of *The Truth About Chronic Pain Treatments: The Best and Worst Strategies for Becoming Pain Free*, which she wrote based on her work as a health care provider working with pain patients, and her own experience with chronic pain.

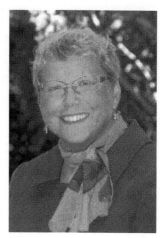

Cindy discovered the mind-body connection after suffering from severe, disabling back pain for three years. She became a Licensed Clinical Social Worker and nationally-certified biofeedback practitioner.

For 25 years, Cindy has helped people improve their emotional and physical well-being through her private practice near Albany, NY. She recently launched The Alternative Pain Treatment Directory as an additional resource for those struggling with chronic pain.

Wayne: Cindy Perlin is certified in biofeedback, a chronic pain survivor, and author of the book, *The Truth About Chronic Pain Treatments: The Best and the Worst Strategies for Becoming Pain Free*. Cindy, thank you for doing this. We're going to start by going back to the beginning in your life. Where did you grow up and what was your childhood like?

Cindy: I started out in The Bronx in New York City, and then lived on Long Island. The city was getting a little challenging as a place to live, so we moved to Long Island when I was 13. Eventually I came up to Albany, New York, where I've now lived for 39 years, so I've been here a while.

Wayne: You migrated into the field of social work. What was the reason for this?

Cindy: I started as an English major in college, because I loved to read. But when I got to college, I realized that what I really liked about literature was what made people tick and that exploration. So I changed to psychology, and I wanted to do something with that, so I went into social work. I was a caseworker in foster care for a couple years. .

Wayne: When did you start biofeedback to help people with pain?

Cindy: I actually was out of commission partway through graduate school, because of an injury. I hurt my back and I was disabled for three years. Biofeedback helped me get better. I kind of stumbled into it, but it really changed my life and got me back to being able to function again.

I took a job in an administrative position and worked at that for quite a few years while I finished my degree, but what really interested me was helping people to heal, especially from chronic pain and chronic illness in general.

Wayne: What are the types of services you now provide with biofeedback?

Cindy: I do psychotherapy and biofeedback. I work with people with all kinds of challenges, whether it's anxiety and depression, chronic pain, or chronic illness. I work with both peripheral and brain wave biofeedback. Peripheral is everything but the brain. It's measuring hand temperature, muscle tension, skin moisture, and respiration rate. Those are all measures that are affected by stress. That's what helped me, hand temperature biofeedback. Then I got into brain wave biofeedback, because there's incredible potential to heal people by changing the way their brain works.

Wayne: So you had personal experience with chronic pain, and were treated with peripheral biofeedback. Now you also use cranial biofeedback in practice. How do you decide which form to use with your patients?

Cindy: I still use both, depending on the circumstances. Peripheral biofeedback is a shorter time frame. People can practice at home. It's less of a commitment. For some things like anxiety and pain, I might start with that and see how people do and then progress to neurofeedback, which requires more frequent sessions and a longer-term commitment. I'll do that if the peripheral biofeedback doesn't help enough.

Wayne: Let's go back to your own journey with disabling back pain. How difficult was that for you?

Cindy: It was pretty awful, because the doctors just wanted to throw drugs at it. They didn't know what was wrong with me. I went to a lot of doctors. They kept giving me different drugs: opiates, muscle relaxers, anti-inflammatories. Some of the drugs are very dangerous. None of them really helped. I was in despair. I went to one doctor who spent a lot of time with me, and seemed to be very compassionate, but who said, "You might have this the rest of your life." I was only 25 and it was agony. I really didn't want to live like that for the rest of my life.

I even started thinking about suicide. Luckily a friend of mine intervened and said, "You've got to read this book." The book was *Anatomy of an Illness*, about a man who laughed his way back to health after experiencing a chronic progressive joint disease. He mentioned biofeedback, so I went and got a treatment. The fact that I had to stumble on it that way almost by accident, that the doctors didn't guide me to it or suggest it, that they knew nothing about it and held out no hope for me, was all very discouraging. That's why I'm so committed to getting the message out now to people with pain that there are options. There are lots of them, not just biofeedback. It's not just about taking drugs. If you want to get better, you have to look at the root cause and you have to address it.

Wayne: Thank you so much for that testimony. One of the reasons for this book is to hear from people and professionals who have suffered with pain, or treat pain, and had to find new ways to achieve successful results. Our traditional medical model does not deal with the root cause of pain or the mind-body approach for solutions. Many patients are just stuck with their situation, and can't move on with their life. They're often demoralized and struggle on. So, thank you for your story.

In your case, what was the root cause that you could identify?

Cindy: I think originally it was a physical injury, because it started when I took up running, trying to get in better shape. As I continued to run, my back hurt more and more. I had these shoe inserts that were made out of hard plastic, and I think that was part of the problem. And then, once I was in pain, I think the stress of being in pain and not seeing an improvement made things worse. Once you have a muscle injury, you're much more susceptible to pain from stress. So it became a cyclical thing. I was stressed and upset about the pain, and I wasn't healing because of that. I needed to get out of that place to get better.

Wayne: Stress is a very real thing for many of us. How was your journey of reducing or reversing it?

Cindy: It was really about going to the psychologist who did biofeedback and finding out that my mind affected my body, because I really didn't know that until I read that book I mentioned, where the author had laughed himself to better health. I didn't understand the physical effect of worrying. I would worry the night before about the next day, and how I was going to get through it. The psychologist explained that that worry was going to make things worse, that I would wake up having already created stress in my body that would exacerbate the pain.

He taught me a very simple relaxation technique. He gave me what you could call a portable biofeedback device. It was actually just a strip that changed color depending on how stressed or relaxed you were. My pain was reduced 50% in one day, because the stress of feeling out of control was gone. Now I had learned there was something I could do to make the pain better. I no longer believed that my body was just attacking me, and there was nothing I could do about it, that it wasn't of my own making, it was this alien part of me that was creating it. That belief was corrected.

That intervention is called "cognitive behavioral therapy", which can be very, very helpful for people in pain. Just connecting their thoughts to what's happening in their body and learning how to monitor and shift thoughts is very important.

Wayne: It was certainly part of my research as a family physician, when I was looking for solutions and ways of helping patients with pain. The cognitive behavioral model and cognitive behavioral techniques are just so important and often so easily done. For example, simple breathing exercises or stopping negative thoughts as they come into your head and replacing them with neutral or positive thoughts. I've had a similar experience with many patients who can take on this type of approach. So, good for you. It's great to hear.

You've written a book about this subject. Could you tell us a little bit about that?

Cindy: The book is really an overview of all the different pain treatments that are out there, conventional and alternative. It goes through the drugs: the opioids, the nonsteroidal anti-inflammatory drugs, and things like gabapentin or neurontin. It looks at the problems with those approaches and with surgical approaches. Then it goes into other kinds of alternative healing: the mind-body approach that we were just talking about, acupuncture, physical therapy, chiropractic, and low-level laser therapy, which is something I had never heard of before I started researching my book. It goes through all these different therapies and talks about the research behind them. It has interviews with patients and practitioners in terms of their experience with the different techniques. So, it's really an overview of what's likely to be helpful and what's not. And of course it also mentions my own experience in healing.

As an outgrowth of my book, I've created a website that does a similar thing. It's at www.paintreatmentdirectory.com. It has lots of articles, it has products, and it has providers that can help with chronic pain.

Wayne: Thank you for sharing that. I will certainly look into that myself and utilize some of your resources. As you move forward, what's the biggest challenge you're facing now?

Cindy: I think because I've set so many goals for myself professionally, that personally it's hard to get enough life/work balance. Professionally, I think there are a lot of challenges. I'm trying to work on the issue that health insurance does not pay for the treatments that help people the most, which I think is a huge problem.

The other part of that is because opioids have been pushed on patients for so long and so many people have become dependent on them, there are so many patients out there who don't believe anything else could help them. They've been so brainwashed that opioids are the best thing for chronic pain. But actually they're one of the worst things, because they might help initially, but over time they make it harder to overcome pain. I hear from people who've been taking opioids for decades, and they're still in terrible chronic pain. They've needed more and more opioids to get the same effect. Their lives are very constricted. They're still in a lot of pain and they're just stuck. Convincing them that something else could work better is very challenging.

Wayne: With this opioid crisis that's upon us in North America, we really do need alternative solutions. Thank you for your work with your book and your website where people can go and find answers for their pain issues.

Just to wrap up, is there anything else you'd like to share that we haven't already discussed?

Cindy: That's a good question. I do think the importance of nutrition should be mentioned. There are many nutritional deficiencies that could cause pain. For instance, omega 3 fatty acids, or vitamin D. You're even farther north than I am. People get very little sun on their skin, which is the main way we make vitamin D. Just a vitamin D deficiency can cause widespread pain. Magnesium is another deficiency. Then there are things we ingest that are not good for us and can cause chronic pain, like aspartame, which is also called NutraSweet, and MSG. Some people are very gluten-sensitive, and even though they might not have the classic gluten Celiac Disease symptoms, they do get pain from gluten.

So I think there are three basics for self-care. One is that mind-body connection, managing stress. The second is moving your body, because if you don't move your body, that's going to create more pain. You have to find the right exercise. The third is diet. If you take care of those three things, most likely you're not going to need a lot of outside intervention.

Wayne: Thank you again for your testimony, for your journey and personal health success, and for using your insights and training to help other people with this very big problem we have on our hands in the medical community.

Chapter 12
KIMBERLY PETREE

Kimberly Petree is a leading Integrative Health Care Practitioner, with more than 22 years experience in women's health and wellness.

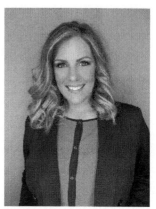

She owns a practice in Alpharetta, Georgia, and also offers both local and international wellness retreats.

Kimberly is also an author of two wellness books, speaker and advocate for Integrative Health and Medicine, and a teacher and chapter leader for the national *Holistic Mom's Network* and *Propel Women's Ministry.*

Wayne: Kimberly Petree is an integrative health specialist who's been helping patients with chronic pain for over 20 years. She performs treatments with Oriental medicine, bioenergetics and also functional neuromuscular therapy. Kimberly, let's begin by going back. Where did you grow up, and what was your childhood like?

Kimberly: I grew up in the New York City area, so childhood was fun. Of course, growing up in that kind of an atmosphere, you were able to do a lot of fun activities and were exposed to many things, exposed to many different cultures. That was my introduction to the world of alternative medicine therapies. It was a fun childhood experience for me.

Wayne: Where did you go to college, and how did you get into the health field?

Kimberly: I went to the New York College of Health Professions, and then I went to International Bioenergetic College. My interest in traditional Chinese medicine was sparked while working as an assistant in a doctor's office with MD's from China. They incorporated modalities like acupuncture, nutrition, and holistic pain therapy with their patients to help them recover from chronic illnesses and metabolic disorders, as well as pain issues. Seeing the results from this model of patient care propelled me into going further into Oriental medicine therapy and the neuromuscular field. Helping people and see the amazing changes in their lives became my passion at this time in my life.

Wayne: Excellent. So what is Oriental medicine therapy?

Kimberly: Oriental medicine therapy is based in the theory of Oriental medicine diagnosis and application. We use the traditional methods of Oriental medicine diagnosis with the tongue and pulse, and then we assess the body on the mind, energetic and spiritual levels, all the levels that Oriental medicine looks at. Then we apply our hands to manipulate the acupuncture points of the body. There's no actual insertion of needles. Instead we use our hands for more sensitivity to things going on in the body. We can feel the energy moving in, through, and around the acupuncture point, and we can feel those energetic changes with our hands to further assess the healing process with the patient.

Wayne: Is that something you develop over time through many years of practice, or is it something that you're naturally gifted with?

Kimberly: I think everyone's different. Some people do just have that innate sensitivity. I know I did when I started, but it definitely develops and gets stronger as you lay your hands on more people. There's something to be said for time put in. You grow your skills and expertise through working with people, and interacting with different personalities and anatomies in both physical and energetic levels.

Wayne: And what is the bioenergetic approach all about?

Kimberly: The bioenergetic approach is the cellular health of the person. It's also looking at the energetic health of the person. It's an incorporation of holistic healing modalities such as Oriental medicine theory, homeopathy and nutritional medicine. The main focus is on cellular health and repairing inside the cells, the extracellular fluid and then building from that point on to create health in the body.

Wayne: Let's say a patient comes in and you decide this is the best approach for them. Take us through an example of how you do an assessment.

Kimberly: If someone comes in and they're experiencing chronic pain, chronic illness, we start off with a full body assessment. I look at the entire body from the outside, and I see what their posture is showing me, where their tightness is, where their imbalances are. I use a program and take a full body image, and show them where their imbalances are in the soft tissue. I explain how these imbalances also affect the neurological and organ system. Then we would look at the inside of the body and see where their deficiencies are in the organs and in the cells, and if it's an energetic deficiency. I use muscle testing to see what supplements are needed to get them started on that healing path. I also incorporate the option for functional lab work to see what their hormonal and nutritional needs are. It's an all-encompassing treatment plan. It's not just one therapy treating everything. I don't believe there's one pill or one therapy that can help everyone across the board. We have to look at the person as an individual and come up with that customized individual approach. That's what we look at, and that's what we try to achieve with integrative and holistic medicine therapies.

Wayne: So once you've done your assessment, and you understand the problem, what treatment modalities do you use?

Kimberly: I start off with postural assessment, muscle testing, functional lab testing and then we move into the actual hands-on therapy time where I typically will start with soft tissue work around the neck. I believe that whatever is happening with your head, whether it's your mental state, stress, or pain, it refers throughout the entire body. I always try to get their head and neck and shoulders relaxed and released of whatever stress and tension is there. If there are any imbalances in there, we work to release the soft tissue to help with imbalance. From there, we continue on to wherever the major pain point is in their body. If it's a knee issue or a back issue, I use the functional neuromuscular work, which is an incorporation of the postural analysis, trigger point therapy, fascia release, activated stretching and so forth. There's a whole plethora of techniques and tools I've incorporated from over 20 years of education and applied skills.

Wayne: This fascinates me. In my own practice I do fascia release with medical needles, and I find this a helpful approach. I'm also aware of the hands-on approach to release fascia with different degrees of pressure or movement, from the subtlest of pressure of touch to the deep tissue massage, like Rolfing.

Say a patient comes in and you're doing a treatment to the neck and upper body. What is actually happening from your perspective? What thoughts are going through your mind as you treat this patient?

Kimberly: What's going through my mind is getting their stress level down. If they're stressed, if they can't control their breathing, and if they can't get into a coherent state, that's really what I'm focused on in the beginning. We want to get that stress down, their coherence level up so they can focus and receive the techniques that are there to help them. That's really what I'm looking to do on that first treatment session. Sometimes it takes more than one time to get them there. It's just getting that stress level down, getting their cortisol levels down, getting the parasympathetic system to relax. Sometimes getting them to just be still is a big achievement for a lot of people, to just be still in their body, in their mind, in their breathing, and to accept the healing that they can receive.

Wayne: As this happens, the patient become more relaxed and the stress levels are dropping, is the body finding its own equilibrium on its healing journey?

Kimberly: That's right. Just like when you're working the fascial system. As you said, when you work the fascial system, it's a very light touch. If you're doing it in response to what they are showing you, it just releases and the body does what it needs to do. It knows where it needs to go. It's the same approach. Like you said, you want to be able to have their equilibrium and their homeostatic level just nice and calm in order to get into those deeper levels of healing. You can't just go in with a hammer and start hammering out areas of pain because that just creates more trauma in the body as well.

Wayne: I've had patients who respond very well to this approach. I can certainly relate to that. Looking ahead, what's the biggest challenge you're facing in your career?

Kimberly: I would say working with people and having them work through their fears. I think a lot of people that come in to see me have a lot of fear. It's fear about, "I don't know what's going to happen to me. I have all these different conditions going on." There's a lot of fear of the unknown and a lot of fear of not knowing the steps to take. My biggest challenge is getting people to work through that fear because it's something they're bombarded with all the time in these different advertisements for different medications, and then they get into the syndrome of, "Oh, I have this, I have that because I'm having these symptoms." Then you have the Googling of symptoms. It just creates a lot of fear in people. My challenge is working through that fear and getting people to realize that the body is made to be healthy and whole, and once you give it the tools it needs, it can achieve that.

Wayne: Yes, moving away from fear toward a more peaceful state that allows the body to heal. Who is an ideal patient for you?

Kimberly: My ideal patient is women around 45 and up. They have usually been through a lot, and usually I'm the last stop. They're experiencing a lot of health issues, whether it's an autoimmune issue or they want to prevent progressing into a further health issue they have. Usually with their health issues, there is a lot of pain, a lot of stress, a lot of anxiety. Those are the areas that I love to work with and help people achieve their health in those areas.

Wayne: What would be the first step you would want these ideal patients to take?

Kimberly: The first step I always have them take is nutritional work. There's always a nutritional component that needs to be addressed in their health issues. I believe if we can't get a hold on having healthy nutrition, there's nothing to sustain the body to progress into a further healing state. For me, it's always nutrition first. Getting hydrated, making sure they're getting in plenty of healthy vegetables coming from a healthy source, and healthy meats, and getting enough protein, enough minerals. All of that is the first step that I take with the patients.

Wayne: I love your approach here. You give a lot of good advice. What is the best advice you have ever received?

Kimberly: It came from someone who has been a doctor for many, many years and is as passionate about helping people as I am. It's hard to be around people you see are suffering and hurting and you want to help. The best advice I have received to help me get through that is you can't help them unless they ask for it. That's been my best advice as a practitioner. You have to let them need the help from you.

Wayne: They have to be ready to receive. Good. Where could people go to learn more about you?

Kimberly: I have my website, kimberlypetree.com, and that's also the name of my Facebook page.

Wayne: Excellent. I'm sure readers will be looking you up, to dive a bit more into what services you provide. Thank you for sharing many different approaches in your integrative healing practice.

Chapter 13

JACOB TEITELBAUM

Jacob Teitelbaum, MD, is a nationally-known expert in the fields of chronic fatigue syndrome, fibromyalgia, sleep and pain.

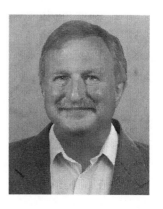

He is the Director of the *Center for Effective CFIDS/Fibromyalgia Therapies* and the Medical Director of the *Fibromyalgia and Fatigue Centers*, in Kona, Hawaii, and the founder of the *Practitioners Alliance Network*.

Dr. Teitelbaum is the author of numerous books including, *The Fatigue and Fibromyalgia Solution, Pain Free 1-2-3: A Proven Program for Eliminating Chronic Pain Now, Three Steps to Happiness Healing Through Joy*, the *Beat Sugar Addition NOW!* series, *Real Cause, Real Cure*, and the iPhone and Android application, *Cures A-Z*. He is also the lead author of four studies on effective treatment for fibromyalgia and chronic fatigue syndrome.

Wayne: Dr. Jacob Teitelbaum is an internal medicine specialist, and the author of many books about pain and health. He's well-known across the world as a guest on Good Morning America, the Dr. Oz show,

Oprah and Friends, CNN, and Fox News Health. It's a great privilege to have him here. Let's dive in and get going.

What led you into medicine?

Jacob: I tend to be pretty empathic. Even as a young child I just wanted to help people overcome all the different kinds of pains, physical and emotional. I grew up in a family of concentration camp survivors. Most of my community had been at Auschwitz and the other camps. That made for a pretty intense childhood. For me it was being a doctor. That's what being a healer was. That was the avenue that was available. I got to experience being on the other side of the white coat in 1975 when I came down with fibromyalgia after a nasty viral syndrome while in medical school. It's funny, the doctors and professors are all well-meaning, but they had no idea. They knew I had a viral infection, the test was clear, but they couldn't identify why I wasn't getting better.

Since I was paying my own way through medical school, that actually left me homeless, sleeping in parks. It was from this experience that I learned what I needed to do to get myself well, and I've spent the last 40 years researching this area. Again, chronic pain, chronic fatigue, fibromyalgia, these are all very treatable, and we're going to teach people how to get well.

Wayne: Wonderful. You trained as an internal medicine specialist. You developed a natural tendency for helping and treating pain because you've experienced fibromyalgia. Please share more about your education.

Jacob: It was ironic. When I was sleeping in parks, it was is if the universe put a holistic homeless medical school sign on my park bench. Health practitioners, MDs, DOs, chiropractors, naturopaths, herbalists, energy workers, all these folks came by. We'd sit, we'd chat, we'd find some pieces of what I needed to learn to recover. Sometimes if they had a pizza with them or something, I ate. I learned more sitting on that park bench of a much wider array than I did even in medical school. Once I recovered and got back to medical school, I was able to really excel. But we didn't even have a name for fibromyalgia back then, or chronic fatigue syndrome. Over time, the pieces of the puzzle came together, because I'm very much a science geek. It's not uncommon for me to go through dozens of studies in a day and tear them apart to see what they really show beyond who's sponsoring the study. I was shocked when I realized that much of what I was being taught in medical school wasn't science. It was pharmaceutical company slick advertising masquerading as science.

The research had so much more to offer than what I was being taught. What I learned in medical school is very helpful, but simply reading the scientific literature has opened a broad new world. Having the pleasure to meet and speak with Dr. Janet Travell, and with other people who have been training with her, opened up a whole new area for me.

Wayne: Okay, let's start with this whole new area of treating pain.

Jacob: It's important to realize there are four domains that need to be addressed for pain. Biophysics, biochemistry, structural, and mind-body all need to be addressed. Medicine does so very poorly. Let's look at the biophysics. What happens when muscles don't have enough energy? If muscles don't have enough energy they're like a spring, they get locked in a shortened position. It takes more energy to stretch the muscle than to contract it. When you don't have enough energy in the muscles, you're going to find they get locked in a shortened position and they hurt. If you have it just locally because of repetitive stress injury, or ergonomics, one local area is getting energy drained, then it's a local pain. When you have a widespread energy crisis in the muscles and throughout the body, then you basically have widespread pain as in fibromyalgia.

To release the muscles means to restore and enhance energy production within the muscle. When you do that, it releases. The tight belly of the muscle when it contracts is a tender knot called a trigger point. If you put a needle in, especially if you turn it, it creates a current. That current is a form of energy, and it will release the muscles. It's interesting, if you map out trigger points and acupuncture points, 70% of them are in overlap, so there's more going out in the area of biophysics.

I remember in medical school they used to call me the ghost because if you walked in the medical library at 2:00, 4:00 in the morning, I'd be there cruising through the stacks, pulling things off, and reading. My routine was to take a journal from 100 years ago, 50 years ago, 20 years ago, and today, and just get perspective over time what had been going on. A hundred years before I was in medical school there was all this research being done by the people who my textbooks were named after. Major neurologists and others in the field, like Professor Guyton and the rest. They were looking at biophysics in a disease that was then called hysterical paralysis, which is now known as multiple sclerosis. There was all this research going on in biophysics and the rest. Then suddenly I could see where it all stopped. These authors all stopped publishing in the area. It was as if, and I suspect this is what happened, the pharmaceutical industry was on the rise, and basically told them if you don't stop looking at that nonsense your funding is gone. You could see, it just all shifted to biochemistry, which is the pharmaceutical industry, which is where the money is.

In the eastern cultures, traditional Chinese medicine and chakra work, the main focus is biophysics because medications are too expensive, and biophysics is cheap. Put simply, acupuncture, chakra, and other systems worked. Where in the west, it was money, money, money, and biochemistry reigned and anything else except for surgery got suppressed. Here we are now in the next part of the cycle, reclaiming the bigger picture. Doctors have taught about medications or surgery, and there's so much more. When you use that whole toolkit, almost all pain can be effectively treated.

Wayne: So trigger point dry-needling releases the muscles by producing a micro current of energy to relax the muscle, and then the patient can mobilize easier and move on to active exercise. Exercise is essential for a healthy body. Let's move on to the second domain of biochemistry you've mentioned. There's nutrition, medications, and there's herbal treatments. What do you suggest for the nutrition approach for healing pain?

Jacob: Let me give one other key concept, that pain is not an outside invader. It's not like an infection. Pain is part of our body's normal healthy monitoring system, saying something needs attention. It's like the oil light on a car's dashboard. Say the oil light goes off, you take it to the tire doctor, and you say this light's annoying. First thing the doctor does is put a band-aid over it, which is like giving Ibuprofen or NSAIDs. It's not surprising then that we see 30,000 to 50,000 U.S. deaths a year from those medications. Don't hear about in the news media in part because who's their biggest advertiser? Well, Ibuprofen is one of them. As a magazine editor once said to the reporters, if you write anything that loses us an advertising account, you're fired. So you don't get to hear about that research.

So the next thing we do in medicine is we try to cut out the oil light. How about if we just put oil in the car? If we give the car what it says it's needing. You put oil in the car, the oil light goes away. Our research has shown if you give the body what it needs, it's perfectly happy and the pain goes away. That's the key thing here. If you're looking at the pain coming from low energy, which is the main thing for muscle pain, our research showed that the SHINE protocol optimizing Sleep, Hormones, Infections, Nutrition, Exercise as able, optimizes energy production and the pain gets much less and often goes away. In fact, the majority of people in our study no longer qualified as having fibromyalgia by the end of the study. The P value was less than .001 versus placebo. A dramatic effect when you do this.

Looking at N for nutrition, start with the simple things. I like a vitamin powder because I don't like people taking handfuls of pills. With a powder I can get 50 pills worth of nutrients in one drink. There's one called the *Energy Revitalization System* vitamin powder, which makes it very easy for people. Other energy nutrients are important, such as Ribose. In two of our studies D-Ribose increased energy production an average of 61%, which was remarkable. We actually have a SHINE Ribose, but there are all kinds of Ribose out there. Just use the powder, because why take 30 pills when you can take a 5g group of powder? Just add it to water or your coffee or tea. Coenzyme Q-10, Acetyl L carnitine are also helpful. Magnesium and B vitamins are already in the vitamin powder, but those two are critical. You do that, and even those simple things can dramatically decrease pain and increase energy.

I used to live on the Chesapeake Bay in Annapolis, Maryland. Now I live in Hawaii, so life's getting better and better. But I remember in Maryland one day I was walking along the city dock and I saw this guy eyeing me from across the street. I looked at him and he's eyeing me. Suddenly he tears across the street through traffic, runs over to me, puts me in a big bear hug and lifts me off the ground. I said, "Who are you? And we haven't even had a first date yet, put me down." He said, "I'm sorry. You're Dr. Teitelbaum aren't you?" I said yes. He said, "Well I had this chronic back pain for decades. Nobody could do anything about it. I took the energy revitalization system vitamin powder and my back pain went away." The high dose B vitamins, magnesium, these are critical for energy production of the muscles. Sometimes it's that simple.

Then you want to keep sugar in the diet low. I have my sweet tooth and I'm a chocoholic, but you don't want to do sodas and juices that have 3/4 teaspoon of sugar per ounce. If you have widespread things like fibromyalgia or low blood pressure, there's a good chance you have orthostatic intolerance. That means when you stand up, blood rushes to your legs and you get brain fog and tired. In that case, increasing salt and water intake is a very good idea. If, as they say, you drink like a fish and pee like a racehorse, it suggests that you're having a deficiency of the hormone called ADH, a vasopressin that holds onto water. That's very common in these processes.

Wayne: Thank you for these tips on nutrition. Your books have a lot more information for people to utilize. Now what about herbal treatments for chronic pain?

Jacob: The herbals can be very helpful, but it's part of the biochemistry. Medications, herbals, and nutrients. If I was on a desert island and could only take one herbal with me for pain, it would be a mix called Curamin. This is a mix of a highly absorbed curcumin.

Most are not. What you get in one of a highly absorbed curcumin would take seven pills of pure curcumin and 350 pills of turmeric. This is a case where I have my people specifically take this one. The Curamin is a mix of highly absorbed curcumin, Boswellia, DLPA, and Nattokinase, all four of those together. It's funny, when I first tried it with folks I figured there would be some synergy. But I had people whose pain wasn't being helped by morphine, and their pain went away after six weeks on Curamin. That's my favorite.

There's another herbal mix called End Pain. It's a mix of willow bark, Boswellia, and cherry, which is excellent. The two are synergistic. I would use topical comfrey. Comfrey has both healthy and unhealthy components. A form called Traumaplant only has the healthy components. Don't take it by mouth, use the topical cream. The list goes on from there, but those are my favorites.

Wayne: Excellent. Then medications. Which medications are you prescribing for chronic pain?

Jacob: There are over 30. It depends on the type of pain. I will use the NSAIDs, which is like Ibuprofen, but not very often, because of a couple head-on studies. The Curamin was studied against Celebrex on arthritis and rheumatoid arthritis, and it was more effective. Instead of side effects, you get side benefits. Going back to SHINE, it's not just a matter of using medications and herbals to treat the pain. I'm going to address sleep, because if you don't sleep the pain doesn't go away. It's that simple. People often have poor sleep with their chronic pain.

For sleep, you need to look at initiating sleep and maintaining sleep. Some people have trouble falling asleep, some have trouble staying asleep. Many have both. To fall asleep, the medications Ambien, which is Zolpidem, and its cousins, are the most effective. At lower doses we don't see much addiction, but we will with doses over 12.5 milligrams a day. But the main problem is, when you stop it you get rebound insomnia from hell, so you don't stop it suddenly. You gradually wean. Trazodone 25 to 50 milligrams, Cyclobenzaprine 2.5 to 5 milligrams, Tizanidine or Zanaflex 2 to 4 milligrams at bedtime. The Zanaflex and the Trazodone can also be taken through the day for pain, but not the Trazodone, the Flexeril or the Zanaflex. As long as you use low dosing, the side effects are usually minimal for most people. 2.5 milligrams is the optimal dose for the Flexeril Cyclobenzaprine, and then the Zanaflex 2 to 4 milligrams. If you increase the dosage and side effects appear, cut back the dosage or don't use that drug.

In my books, and in the phone app, we talk about literally dozens and dozens of both prescriptions and the natural options. But again, if you treat sleep, that's one of the most effective pain medications you can be giving. People do better with a low dose. There are herbal mixes. My favorite is called Revitalizing Sleep Formula. There's Terrific ZZZZ's. I've found a sustained release melatonin you can get on Amazon called Dual Spectrum by Nature's Bounty. It has an immediate and sustained release, which works much better than most melatonins. Even a hot Epsom salt bath at bedtime, two cups of Epsom salts in a tub of hot water and you soak.

It doesn't have to be expensive. I don't think anything I've mentioned is expensive. It's all cheap, which is why I'm guessing that most doctors have never heard about these, or at least not much. They hear about the newer more expensive medications. Because as the bank robber said when asked why he robs, banks, "That's where the money is."

Wayne: Let's go back to the four domains of healing you mentioned. The third was structural. Where does manipulation fit in for treating chronic pain?

Jacob: You're going to see a couple key areas. One, the muscle shortening is the most common cause and common missed cause of chronic pain in North America. What you'll see is if you release the muscle, the pain goes away. Now we've talked about using dry-needling to put energy in, but you can also use what's called ischemic compression. Your push, maybe a good amount of pressure on the belly of the muscle for 45 seconds until it hurts so much that the person wants to punch you. But that also is a form of energy. In this case electric energy where you're putting energy into the muscle. But more importantly, I just don't think it's able to hold the tightness in response to that, so the muscle releases. Whether you're doing chiropractic or osteopathic manipulation, or myofascial release, or I could give you hundreds of names of different kinds of things that all basically say release muscle, the pain will go away.

The problem is if you don't treat the root cause, the low energy, the ergonomic thing, with your hip heights being uneven or whatever, muscle is going to go right back to shortened position. You'll feel better for a couple hours or days, but you haven't gotten the root cause. My friend Hugh Gilbert does a process that you might want to look into called *Kinetic Chain Release*. Just do a search online. Because once the muscles get stuck in the shortened position, the joints also lose their range of motion. Until you do a passive stretch to get that range of motion back, it cases pain and dysfunction. He does a simple thing takes about 10 to 15 minutes. We can go through each of the key joint areas and release those joints.

That's the beginning thing. You've now set the body up where you've released the old tightening in the joints themselves, around the joints. But the next thing, which I think is a massive area that's coming over the horizon now, is fascial release. As a physician, we never really talked about fascial. There was some dead tissue that was ignored. Then over the years it seemed more like a fibrous band of tissue that kind of holds the muscles into their alignment. You could use things like raw finger things where you've got to stretch those fascia to help reset and rebalance so they're the same length on each side. But what's coming out now is, these fascia are not dead fibrous tissue. This is a very active dynamic system of the body.

We've heard about the "fight or flight" reaction. A bear is chasing you, so you either run or climb, or fight if you're cornered. But in addition to "fight or flight," there's also "freeze." What happens when you can't run and you can't hide? Say you're in your car and you look in your rear view mirror and you see this truck getting ready to plow into you. You can't run and you can't hide. The third thing is freeze. The fascia tightens everything up almost like a suit of armor to protect you in the face of the impact, or injury, or whatever it happens to be. It can also be physical or sexual abuse, whatever you can't run from or fight.

Now freeze is a very healthy system. But you need to unfreeze. Most animals know how to release the freezing. The standard way of doing that is the body goes through this trembling kind of a thing and shakes it off. It's kind of like a football player or a rugby player who gets slammed by 800 pounds of people on the other side. What does the coach say when they guy's spread out on the ground? "Shake it off." This is where that comes from. Because it's the signal to release the fascia. Animals will do that naturally after stress. Anybody's who a zookeeper or game tender has seen that. But humans feel silly doing it so we suppress it. Because of that we hold on to layer after layer after layer of trauma, some building up for lifetimes.

There's a wonderful book called *Waking the Tiger* by Dr. Peter Levine. He talks about a simple, easy technique you can do on your own. When you feel your body going through this trembling thing, let it happen. You'll feel almost like a Novocain numbness has lifted from you. Each one, there will be another wave that comes off. If you're around people you don't know and you don't want to look foolish, suppress it. But if you're with your spouse or friends, explain to them what it is, or just let it happen. This is a natural process and can help the fascial release so the muscles can release and you can begin the healing process.

Wayne: I really appreciate this insight from your perspective, because that's something I've come to realize myself in the last couple years. With my trigger point injection technique, literally freeing the fascia with the penetration of soft tissues with medical needles of increasing gauge size, I've found better outcomes with my patients which are backed up by audit results. I completely connect with what you're saying.

It's interesting that my dog trainer taught me about the stress response in dogs 10 years ago. Dogs shake the stress away. I see my dogs doing the shake dance every day! I've also read another book by Dr. Levine, *In An Unspoken Voice*, which covers similar principles of stress in the body and how to heal. It's fantastic to be talking with you about all this.

Now let's move on to the fourth domain, the mind-body work and the role of feelings. We are not a machine. We are human beings with emotions, thoughts, physical body and a spirit. They all interconnect. This is what I teach my patients every day. Let's talk about how that actually works out in the chronic pain state.

Jacob: In my experience as a physician for more than 40 years, I've found the body very often is a metaphor for what's going on in the psyche and the spirit. If people feel unsupported, they may have back pain.

Multiple sclerosis tends to be people with repressed rage, which is why they're so sweet. Ovarian cancer, hopeless personality. If we have feelings and we don't express them, they will often get buried in the muscles. That's why when you get a massage it's not uncommon for people to have old feelings bubble to the surface. It's called muscle memory.

I treat people from all over the world with fibromyalgia, and we'll often do it by phone because they're too ill to travel. But once you've cleared the biochemistry, if you don't also clear the underlying psychodynamic, which is what your body was trying to achieve through the illness, they're not healed. You have to treat the whole thing.

If you think of fibromyalgia being an energy crisis using one model of pain, what's the psychodynamic we see? We talk about multiple sclerosis being repressed rage. In fibromyalgia it's being unable to say no. We tend to be overachieving people pleasers, who try to be all things to all people and take care of everybody but ourselves. We're afraid to say no to avoid losing approval. That's the psychodynamic for many people. So what do you do? Number one, you ignore your brain, which is just going to feed back to you what you've been taught you should do to get approval. The church, and synagogue, and media, and schools, everybody is telling you that you should make *them* happy and see how things feel.

Say you're walking down the street and you see Mrs. Smith, who chairs the committee of a thousand ways to waste everybody's time, walking down the street the other way. And you notice that everybody is ducking into the alleys except the person with fibromyalgia. They're like a deer in the headlights. If Mrs. Smith comes up to you and says they need you to chair a subcommittee, in a way that will make you want to tear your eyeballs out and run screaming, and she barfs up all this emotional stuff on you, what do you do? Your gut is screaming, "No, run!" Everybody else says no. But what does the person with fibromyalgia say? "Okay."

That's a recipe for an energy crisis. Doctor's orders, when people are asking you to do things that don't feel good, if you're not going to get arrested or be homeless for not doing it, say no. If they say, "But I need you," and all their emotional stuff, tell them the doctor said no and you're following your doctor's advice. They'll usually find somebody else to suck dry.

If I had to give the one simple thing for the mind-body component, it's see how things feel. If they feel good, they're authentic to you, go with them. If they don't feel good, just shift your attention and say no. Don't fight them or shift your attention to them, move onto something else. That's the brief version.

Wayne: Yes, I know researchers at the HeartMath Institute in California study heart-based meditation techniques. Their research shows the more we can live in our happy place, living a heart-centered life with compassion, caring, gratitude and appreciation, the more we heal our bodies. Our heart is programing our brain, and I believe the whole body, through emotions or chemical proteins called neuropeptides. HeartMath has shown the human heart contains 40,000 neurites, or nerve cells, that make up "a little brain" in the heart which is directly connected to brain. This new information is generally unknown in the medical community, but this amazing research, started in 1991, further proves the mind-body connection.

Thank you for going through these four pillars of healing for chronic pain. Looking at yourself now, what are the biggest challenges you're currently facing in your career?

Jacob: For me, it's not so much a challenge as much as the next fun thing. It's almost like a Rosetta stone or a missing link between the immune system and the autonomic system. We thought these were two separate boxes, but we're finding they're intricately related. Whether looking at small fiber neuropathy from the autonomic dysfunction, central desensitization behind it, as initiating process of it, or the orthostatic intolerance, POTS, NMH, low blood pressure issues. We're finding that most of the people we're seeing with the autonomic dysfunction, blood pressure, gut issues, are also having deficiencies of certain immune factors. It's called IgG3 and then IgG1 secondarily. There's so much more available now to treat.

I want to mention one other thing for the biophysics. There's a technique called *Frequency Specific Microcurrent*. It's developed by Dr. Carolyn McMakin, who's a chiropractor in Portland, Oregon. It can be very, very helpful. If you're looking for a biophysics technique beyond the traditional chakra, acupuncture kinds of things, it's very powerful and well worth looking into.

The other thing I would look at, is each kind of pain is like a different warning light on a car's dashboard. Each is asking for different things. If you would like, I'm happy to go through and take each of the most common kinds of pain, see what it's saying, and see what the body is asking for.

Wayne: Yes, let's do that. Let's start with back pain.

Jacob: Okay, back pain most often is going to be muscular. There will be some arthritic component in some, but the research has shown that the X-rays show virtually nothing with the back pain unless there is a very specific neurologic deficit out of sight of a specific change in the disc that is the area of the pain. Because we are an upright species. Everybody has normal wear and tear on their spine. There was actually a study looking at people with back pain. They did X-rays and MRIs for people with back pain and those without. First they showed the ones with back pain to radiologists, who said, "This is just horrible", disease, minefield, all that stuff. Then, being troublemakers kind of like me, they took the X-rays of people with no pain, showed them to the radiologists, and lied, saying these people had pain, and got the same responses. "I'm amazed they can walk", that sort of thing. Then they basically put them all up on the screens in front of a group of radiologists and said, "Pick out the ones with pain and the ones without." They couldn't do it any better than chance.

People need to realize if they have back pain and normal wear and tear, which may be read as horrible disc disease on their X-ray, the X-ray is meaningless. Most often it's going to be muscle pain, so we use the SHINE principle. First of all, you want to make sure the hip heights are even. Not the leg lengths, that's a separate thing. I put a person in front of me, both sitting and standing, with their feet together. I put my hands on top of the crest on top of the hip and I make sure they're even. If one of them is even a centimeter off, that's going to throw the whole back out of alignment and trigger a lot of back pain. I find sometimes a simple $15 heel lift makes the pain go away.

Simple structural things, like if you carry a wallet in your back pocket, you've created this incredible curvature of your spine. Put it in your front pocket instead. Instead of taking the money all out and giving it to surgeons, just move it to your front pocket. Earlier I talked about the Curamin doing well in a study for arthritis. It also did well in a study for back pain. And the End Pain was twice as effective as NSAIDs in a head-on study for back pain. You want to give these six weeks to work. They can be used together. They can be used with any pain medications. Then if there is a refractory persistent back pain once you've treated the muscle components, and the X-ray shows an area of specific disc, then when surgery is done for the right reasons it tends to go very well and without post-surgery syndrome and all of the other things. It's mostly when people have it done for the wrong reasons, that they seem to get problems after surgery. But surgery should be the last resort after the other things are done.

Wayne: Okay. What about neck pain?

Jacob: Neck pain can be very similar to the back pain. It's just a different part of the back. The hip heights being off will throw the shoulders. If one hip is higher, that shoulder will be lower, and everything is now out of balance trying to walk and maintain that. So it's the same simple things we talked about. But for the neck pain, ergonomics is a major thing. If you're sitting at a computer with no support under your elbow or wrist, it is the same as walking around for hours a day. Do it for 45 minutes and see where you hurt. You want to make sure your elbows and wrists are supported when you're at your work station or computer. Major, major thing. Also, that your feet are resting flat on the floor.

Simple structural ergonomics in that case, but also emotional. If you find you're having a lot of stress and you're internalizing it, you're clenching your jaw. Do you find you're tender? Go an inch below the middle of the ear, and put a finger inside your mouth, thumb on the outside, and go all the way back to where the cheek goes to getting thick, that's where the muscles are for the jaw joint. If you squeeze them between your fingers and they hurt like hell and reproduce your pain, don't let anybody cut on you. There are topical creams or prescription mixes that are wonderful, compounding pharmacies can make them, that you can put over the jaw muscles. You can also use a bite guard at night. But addressing the jaw joint can be an important area for neck pain as well.

Wayne: Thank you for this insight. Compounding pharmacies are wonderful for making creams and gels for topical application of combination medications for the mouth and skin for pain. Family doctors can prescribe these. I find compounding pharmacies very helpful for educating patients as well.

What about migraines? I find there's a huge crossover between migraine headache, tension headaches, neck pain, and TMJ pain. What's your advice for migraines?

Jacob: It is a spectrum, so you want to take a look. With the migraines you can think of it as an energy crisis in the blood vessels, and their ability to contract and relax. That's a gross over-simplification, but here are the simple things you can do. If you look at our Cures A to Z app, vitamin B2 Riboflavin 400 milligrams a day has been shown to decrease migraine frequency by 69% after six weeks. Magnesium and Vitamin B-12 decrease migraine frequency. Petadolex, which is the form of butterbur I would use, also decreases migraine frequency. It can be used both for acute migraines and for prevention. But for prevention, addressing food allergies is important. The app will talk about the most common foods that trigger migraines. An elimination diet for just those foods for six weeks can help.

In most cases, these simple things will give a dramatic relief for migraine headaches. For acute migraines, the Triptans are helpful, but Excedrin Migraine is just as effective as the Triptans in head-on studies. Why don't doctors hear about that? Excedrin is 35 cents, Triptan $50 a pill. Which one do you have the drug reps coming in and teaching you about? No Excedrin Migraine reps, and I'm betting no Vitamin B-2 reps. The conferences we go to, who's being paid to be up on the podium? Professors that are on the payroll of the drug companies of what they're talking about. Well meaning, but it's just a sad truth of how doctors get education these days.

The most effective way to eliminate an acute migraine, short of decapitation, which I don't recommend even though many sufferers probably feel like they'd like it at the time, is intravenous magnesium. One gram over 15 minutes. It's been shown in two double-blind studies to eliminate 85% of migraines within 45 minutes, and that migraine will not come back for that episode. Why don't most doctors know about that research? Because the magnesium costs five cents.

Wayne: Wow.

Jacob: You'll find, if you're able to do infusions in your practice, use one gram over 15 minutes and migraines will be gone 85% of the time. Now we will see refractory migraines. Usually those are severe food allergies that aren't being addressed, or commonly a fluctuation in the estrogen and progesterone level is triggering it. You can tell that's the case because it happens mostly around a woman's menses, or ovulation. For that, giving an estrogen patch through the month and the bioidentical progesterone, such as Prometrium. I don't use the creams for that because you get the highs and lows with the creams. I'll use the patch because you get the stable level. I'll change the patch a day or two early so you don't get that end of patch drop-off. That will often help the migraines dramatically.

These are the things your body is saying that it needs in these settings. Address food allergies, address the nutritional deficiencies. Give the body what it needs for the blood vessels to stabilize. Migraines are not hard to treat in most cases. I do have one woman that I'm still looking, but most of the time, I give the vitamin powder and the migraines go way down after six weeks because it has the magnesium and B-2 in it.

Wayne: Thank you for that. That's very insightful, and there's some new information for me there. What about rotator cuff traumas, injuries, and tears?

Jacob: Most often these are going to be repetitive stress injuries. Or, again, it can be from the ergonomics at your computer and those kinds of things. But you're looking at tendon information. You have the issues of the tendonitis and other supportive tissues, including fascial. Of course you want to do the range of motions to keep them from freezing, but what I really like for that is the pain creams. Again, if you have a good compounding pharmacy, you ask them for the pain cream for tendonitis, they'll know. It's just like a Scottish grandmother. They'll all have their own recipe for haggis, but all of them will be good. Each of them will have their own recipe for the pain creams. They'll be a mix of about six or seven different medications. Again, this is an oversimplification, but you find the tender areas that are basically the main areas involved, and you rub the cream over that three times a day. Give it six weeks to eight weeks to see the effect.

Now certainly the End Pain and the Curamin are very helpful to decrease the inflammation in general. We've talked about low energy pain needing SHINE to optimize energy. But for inflammatory pain, the Curamin and the End Pain are very helpful. Those are just outstanding in my practice. I'll use the NSAIDs with them if I need, Ibuprofens and the rest for inflammation. The other thing is fish oil. A big reason we're having the increased inflammation now is excess sugar, excess white flour, and a cut in Omega-

3s in our diet. That's why we see so much more inflammation.

Most fish oils have maybe 10%, 20% Omega-3s. There's not much in them. You're taking seven big pills and then you're burping up rancid oil all day. There's one called Vectomega. You take one pill, it replaces seven fish oil pills. That's what I take each morning myself. Save your sugar budget for the stuff you really love. Go for quality, not quantity. Cut out sodas, cut out fruit juices. Vegetables juices are okay. Fruits are okay too. But if you have 16 ounces of orange juice, that's 12 teaspoons of sugar. You'd have to eat eight oranges to get that. You want to eat eight oranges, knock yourself out. Most people won't.

Wayne: Excellent. We've covered several body areas and specific inflammatory pain. What about neuropathic pain and CRPS or Complex Regional Pain Syndrome?

Jacob: For neuropathic pain, lipoic acid 300 milligrams twice a day. Giving lipoic acid 600 up to 750 milligrams, even two to three times a week in the beginning, is very helpful in diabetic neuropathy and other kinds of neuropathies. Then you take it to once a month. Just want to be watching, have some D50, some sugar for IV in case they drop their blood sugar. But that along with lipoic acid 300 milligrams, even 600 milligrams if their stomach tolerates it, twice a day.

Acetylcarnitine one gram three times a day for two months or so, and then you can drop it down to one gram a day. Multivitamin powder because you don't want too much B-6, but up to 45 milligrams is optimal. You want the B-12, you want the magnesium, you want the host of other nutrients that can be helpful, so the Energy Revitalization vitamin powder has all of that.

Then for medications, you want things that are specific for neuropathy. Advil and codeine don't work very well. I will note something as an aside because right now the U.S. government has declared a war on people in pain. Basically trying to figure they're all junkies on codeine, and make them feel like drug addicts every time they need the prescription, and arrest the doctors that are giving it. Let me make two simple statements. One, chronic pain is more toxic than the narcotics when used properly. And two, most pain can be relieved without narcotics, but those who need it, need it. Just to add a little voice of balanced sanity to that whole political debate.

But I want to finish with CRPS. I still remember when I was about your age and early in pain practice, a woman came in. She had seen every rheumatologist. She had a joint and knee aspiration. She developed CRPS of the leg. I was pretty good at pain, even at that point in my career, but I had never been taught anything about CRPS. She said she was going to have her leg amputated. I told her that's not going to make the pain go away, and I couldn't help her. So she had the leg amputated. She came back to me afterward, and the pain was still there. We now have a lot that's very helpful for CRPS. CRPS has finally joined the ranks of other chronic pain conditions that can be effectively treated. There's intravenous bisphosphonates. Absolutely take low dose Naltrexone 3 to 4.5 milligrams at nighttime. There's intravenous ketamine, and topical ketamines. There's a whole host of things.

Anyone who would like, can email me at fatiguedoc@gmail.com. If you have fibromyalgia, I'll send you information on that. If you have CRPS, ask for the CRPS information and I'll send it along.

Wayne: Thank you so much, Dr. Teitelbaum. This interview has been very informative. I've learned a lot from you. Thank you for sharing your time and your knowledge.

Chapter 14
JEFFREY WASSERMAN

Jeffrey Wasserman, MD, has practiced pain management in Dallas, Texas for more than 20 years. He has pioneered several advanced interventional therapies to relieve chronic pain for his patients.

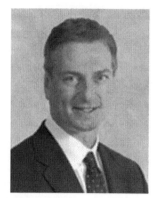

Dr. Wasserman is a specialist in minimally invasive disc healing therapies and spine implants for chronic pain.

He is also a board-certified anesthesiologist in pain management, and a Diplomat of the *American Board of Pain Medicine*. Dr. Wasserman was named one of the Best Doctors in Dallas by *D Magazine*.

Wayne: Dr. Jeff Wasserman is a pain specialist who has practiced in Dallas, Texas for over 20 years and pioneered several advanced interventional therapies to relieve chronic pain for his patients. Dr. Wasserman, thank you for doing this. Let's start with where you grew up, and how you ended up in Dallas.

Jeff: I grew up in Northern New Jersey, a little bit outside Newark in a small town called Maplewood. Two brothers, family dog, mother, father, the usual stuff. I went to Columbia High School there. I went to Lafayette College in Pennsylvania, where I majored in biology. That got me into Penn State University for medical school, because it was pretty close at Hershey, Pennsylvania. While I was there, I was doing research in anesthesia and kind of fell in love with it. So then I did an anesthesia and pain management residency at Massachusetts General, which is the main Harvard teaching hospital in Boston.

I completed that in 1991, and then I stayed on staff with the Harvard teaching hospital in Cambridge. Three years later I moved to Dallas. I met my wife here, and here I stay. We have two kids.

Wayne: Wonderful. So what was it that made you decide to go into anesthesiology or pain management?

Jeff: I actually got into healthcare at the age of 16, when I was a volunteer with a first aid squad up in New Jersey, and immediately knew that's what I wanted to do long term. I highly recommend that for anybody thinking about going into healthcare. You get to spend some time volunteering and you get to see if it's really right for you.

I never wanted to go into healthcare until that. I did it because I thought it was going to be neat to get trained in CPR and become an EMT. But then I quickly learned this was going to be my career.

I got trained as a paramedic while I was in college and medical school. I flew at a helicopter service while I was in medical school. I thought I wanted to be a trauma surgeon or an emergency room doctor. But as it turned out, the people I met who did that just didn't seem happy with what they did. They were burned out and they didn't recommend going into that for a career. Whereas the anesthesiologists at Penn State were happy. They loved what they were doing. I got to do cardiology, I got to do trauma, I got to do the things I liked about medicine that I thought I wanted to do in the emergency room. I found out I could do it in the operating room. So it just led into that.

Wayne: You're obviously following your passion, you love what you do. So what is the best thing about being in this field?

Jeff: Well, the one thing I always thought about anesthesia and being in the operating room is you just don't have your own patients and people never remember your name. Someone has a surgery, you ask them who their anesthesiologist was, and they have a deer in the headlight look. They really don't know. Even though you're responsible for their life during the few hours of the surgery, people don't remember you.

So I didn't like that aspect of it. I found that doing chronic pain medicine, which I'm board-certified in, in addition to anesthesia, you could get a little bit of everything. I was in the operating room, I was doing anesthesia, and I also had a clinic where I was treating patients with chronic pain. And I like the interaction of the patients. I like having the staff, the medical assistants, the nurse practitioners, all working with me. I like the whole patient management thing and not just being in the operating room seeing somebody for a couple hours and never seeing them again.

Wayne: You've actually pioneered some advanced interventional therapies. Let's talk about that.

Jeff: First let me say I didn't actually develop equipment myself. I work with some companies to help them, such as Medtronic. But from the very beginning, whenever new technologies would come out, my colleague Dr. Lloyd and I would be among the first if not the first providers to actually use them in this area of the country. That includes several newer spinal cord stimulator systems, vertebral cementing procedures, and dorsal ganglion stimulation. I also was one of the first in the area to do stem cell injections. We're just on the cutting edge. We like to be able to offer everything to our patients who really don't have any other options. We want to offer everything we can. Obviously we get trained in it first, and we wouldn't offer anything to anybody we wouldn't do on our families or to ourselves.

Wayne: Very good. Please explain what stem cell injections are. How do they actually work? How do they treat pain?

Jeff: There are several different varieties. One is called a bone marrow aspiration. That's where you place a needle into the pelvic bone and get a sample, which is actually quite easy to do. Then you spin it down in a centrifuge and you get a layer that's a concentrate, which are mesenchymal stem cells. We'll inject them into joints, typically, sometimes tendons, to help not just reduce inflammation, but regrow tissue. This is new cutting edge medicine. I believe in 10 or 20 years, this is going to be the way everything's done, whether it's the spine or the joints. We're not just going to be replacing joints, we're going to be helping people to regrow new cartilage.

There's no doubt that's where the future of medicine is. The problem is right now it's in its infancy. We can get stem cells, but keeping the viability of the stem cells is an issue, and then getting them to do what you want them to do. So I can get stem cells and put them into a joint, but can I make it grow into cartilage? Will it become bone? Will it become fat? We're not at that level yet where we even know what they do, other than we know we get some results. But documenting efficacy and making cells become what we want to do, we're not there yet.

And unfortunately, there are some clinics who oversell. They charge a lot of money for it. They're not covered by insurance. And they promise results they cannot really guarantee and they cannot document. Especially stem cell clinics abroad.

In the United States, for example, it's against federal regulations to take stem cells, manipulate them significantly, whether culturing them or making additives, and then re-injecting them back in the patient. You can only take a patient's own stem cells, quickly manipulate them with a centrifuge, and then re-inject them into the patients. The FDA is okay with that.

But once you start culturing them and growing them, especially on culture mediums that have non-human tissue in them, such as Cal fibroblast, you really get in a realm. You can't document safety with that, nor can you document efficacy, let alone charge somebody $50,000 or so to do that, which is extreme. So people get their cells harvested here in the United States, and then they'll fly abroad to Panama or to the Caribbean and have the cells injected into them there. And honestly, that's dubious at best.

Wayne: Thanks for the insightful information. How does the spinal cord stimulator work for the chronic pain patient?

Jeff: Spinal cord stimulation has been around for over 40 years, but the technology has changed dramatically. When I first started doing this, we used to put external receivers on people. They didn't have a battery implanted in them. The basic theory is gate control theory, just like a TENS unit, but much more advanced. If you put an electrical field over the back of the spinal cord, it blocks pain signals that are transmitted in the back of the spinal cord up to the brain. So you basically block the pain signal to that location. You don't change the patient's pathology, per se, but you do change the way their pain is sensed.

Some of the newer systems even affect the emotional component to pain. For example, if I was to cut your skin in your leg, you don't just say, "Ouch," you say it with emotion. And that emotional component of pain may be just as severe as the sensory component with the depression and anxiety and the hypochondriasis that come along with it.

And the newer systems may not only block the pain transmission, but may also positively affect the affective component, the emotional component of pain. So we do a trial of the systems first. We'll place one or two leads into the spinal column, which is done through a needle with a local anesthetic. It's an outpatient procedure that takes just 15 to 30 minutes or so.

We put some tape on the back, and we put a little power source on the patient. They go home with it, and they go about their usual activity. They live with it. They see what it does to control their pain, improve their functioning, and how it affects the use of opiates and other analgesic medications. They usually come back and see us after a week or so. If they have very significant results, it shouldn't be subtle, it should be a very obvious positive result, then we'll implant one of these systems into the patient a week or two later with an implanted battery that's rechargeable. And some of the systems are now MRI compatible as well, so they can have MRIs once they have this system implanted, and they can have that for the rest of their lives if it works well for them.

Wayne: Wow. Thank you for that. What about spine implants?

Jeff: You're probably referring to the Supereon implants. They're little titanium implants that go between the spinous processes of the lower back. So for people who suffer from spinal stenosis that hasn't responded to more conservative therapy, such as physical therapy, medications, and even simple injections, and if they're not a good surgical candidate, then we can implant these devices into the spine in a position where the nerves are not compressed for people's spinal stenosis. Now they can get long-term relief, especially of the pain shooting into their legs, what we call neurogenic claudication that happens with ambulation. So they're able to function much better after the devices. We've had very good results with that. It's a very impressive device so far.

Wayne: Can you share a recent case where spinal implants were used and the benefits found? Obviously keeping confidentiality in mind.

Jeff: Here's one example. I have a patient who's around 70 years old, and she's been in my practice for a long time. She got spinal stenosis at two levels, at L3-4 and L4-5 primarily, stenosis meaning compression of nerves inside the spine due to narrowing of the different spaces, either the central canal or the foramen, the outer canals where the nerves leave the spine. She had both, at both those levels.

Her main problem was back pain radiating into the legs when she would walk more than about 100 feet or so. So she was able to function, but she wasn't able to ambulate, walk around, go shopping, or do the things she wanted to do without having to rest minute or two.

We had treated her medically for years with different medications. She had done physical therapy, chiropractic manipulation. She'd had epidural steroid injections, maybe one or two every year, and got results. I believe we even tried spinal cord stimulation on her. It just didn't work for her, so she never had it implanted. So I offered her the device after getting an MRI scan and getting some flexion/extension X-rays to be sure there was no instability in her spine.

I implanted the device about six months ago. Not only is her pain at rest better, but she's able to now shop and walk several times around the block. So she's able to function better, lose weight, and her lifestyle has changed dramatically.

At the end of the day, what we're all about is not treating pain, per se, but improving the quality of life for the patient. And the main thing of that is how well they're functioning, and can we get them off pain medications that are sedating, cause depression, or have other untoward side effects?

Wayne: Thank you for that excellent case history. What's the biggest challenge you're facing right now?

Jeff: It's a tough time right now to practice medicine in the United States, not so much from the regulatory point of view, but how insurance coverage affects being able to do things in your patients that you want to do. It's very difficult. Remember, we deal in chronic pain patients, so they don't come to us first. They've been through the mill. They've been through several doctors, their primary care physician, and often several other specialists, by the time they get to us.

We're doing pretty novel treatments, and novel treatments aren't liked by the insurance companies. Many of the things we do or we know we can do that will work are considered investigational or experimental, and they're just not covered by insurance. And that's going to become more and more common. The insurance companies are tightening down. They're for-profit businesses, for the most part, so they're worried about making a profit, and many times that doesn't work in the best interest of the patient. Especially when you talk about worker's compensation or those types of systems where nothing can get done. It takes months to get anything pre-authorized. The patients are frustrated. We're frustrated for them. So that's the most negative thing.

But there are positive things happening, too. We talked about regenerative medicine procedures, such as stem cells. I think less reliance upon opiate medications is a positive thing. I think patients are really buying into that. They're seeing it on the news. They know the problem. So I find it much easier these days to wean patients down or off their opiates than a couple years ago, where people really relied upon those as a crutch. Now they are familiar with the danger after the CDC report in 2016.

So there are both negatives and positives these days.

Wayne: Excellent. Last question, what's the best advice you've ever received?

Jeff: To believe in myself. I also have a master's of business, and I'll tell you, the best thing about doing that is you learn about yourself. You learn about your strengths and your weaknesses. You learn to play to your strengths. You know where your weaknesses are. And there are some weaknesses you can't overcome. You just have to accept them and say, "That's me and that's who I am, so let me rely upon my strengths." But that translates into the way you are with patients as well, and your patience with them, and treating everybody the way you'd want to be treated and just being polite. Just believing in myself has allowed me to be a better practitioner.

Wayne: Wonderful. Where could people go to learn more about you or your services?

Jeff: Well, there is my website. It's www.vitalpain.com. Our practice is called *Vital Pain Care.* On the site you can learn about Dr. Lloyd and myself and what we do. We have three clinic locations, in Central Dallas, Addison, and Forney, Texas. So we're focused throughout the Metroplex. We accept all insurances, and we're here to help.

Wayne: Thank you, Dr. Wasserman, for your insights and your service to your population.

CLOSING THOUGHTS

I hope you got as much out of reading these interviews as I did conducting them. These experts and medical professionals shared a wealth of knowledge, and amazing insights.

There's a very important common thread to all these interviews. It's that you don't have to let chronic pain keep you from living your life. Even if you've given up hope of ever getting the relief you need. *There are options that you haven't heard about yet.*

I've been successfully treating people for pain for many years now, and I'm still learning new methods. I'm constantly offering my patients new approaches to treat pain.

As I said earlier in this book, my mission is to help 100 million people live pain free. One of the ways I'm doing that is by teaching other doctors and medical practitioners my scientific holistic approach, which treats both the body and the mind. My patients get pain relief, along with the belief that they can and will get their lives back. They're eliminating or reducing chronic pain, once and for all.

If you'd like to learn more chronic pain solutions follow my podcast on iTunes. It's called *Pain Solutions for the 21st Century.* Or follow my blogs on my website at www.waynephimister.com. If you're here in the Vancouver area and would like to see how I can help you get the pain relief you need, my contact information is at the bottom of this page. My website has the locations of my clinics.

Pain doesn't have to rule people's lives. Relief is out there. I hope you'll join me on this journey of hope.

Dr. Wayne Phimister
2309 McCallum Road
Abbotsford, BC, Canada
V2S 3N7
Phone: 604-850-2511
Fax: 604-850-2581
Email: wayne@waynephimister.com
Website: waynephimister.com

NOTES

NOTES

NOTES

Printed in Great Britain
by Amazon